Seized

Seized

Eve LaPlante

AN AUTHORS GUILD BACKINPRINT.COM EDITION

AN AUTHORS GUILD BACKINPRINT.COM EDITION

Published by iUniverse.com, Inc.

For information address:
iUniverse.com, Inc.
620 North 48th Street, Suite 201
Lincoln, NE 68504-3467
www.iuniverse.com

Originally published by HarperCollins

HarperCollins books may be purchased for educational, business,
or sales promotional use. For information, please write:
Special Markets Department, HarperCollins Publishers,
Inc., 10 East 53rd Street, New York, NY 10022.

Designed by George J. McKeon

ISBN: 0-595-09431-7

Printed in the United States of America

To Virginia W. LaPlante

Few of us are not in some way infirm, or even diseased; and our very infirmities help us unexpectedly.

—William James
The Varieties of Religious Experience

Contents

Preface

Temporal lobe epilepsy is a common neurological disorder that illuminates the relationship between body and mind. The most widespread form of epilepsy among adults, TLE affects roughly one million Americans; by some estimates, another one million sufferers in this country are undiagnosed. The seizures of TLE consist of bizarre hallucinations, strange feelings, and involuntary actions that often resemble the symptoms of psychiatric disease. In addition to these seizures, the disorder is linked with personality change: between seizures many people with TLE are intensely emotional, deeply religious, and compelled to write or draw. In such famous sufferers as Dostoevsky, Tennyson, and Lewis Carroll, these traits may have contributed to lasting works of art. Because of the disorder's links with psychiatric disease and personality change, the study of TLE holds clues to the physiological bases of mental illness, normal human behavior, and creativity.

I learned of TLE in 1984, from a friend, an artist in his thirties. For years he had experienced threatening mental states that had driven him to isolate himself, attempt suicide, and spend months at psychiatric hospitals, where his doctors had suspected psychiatric disease. In 1983 a doctor finally recognized his symptoms as seizures and told him that his problem was actually TLE. Fascinated by the symptoms, the personality changes, and the difficulty of diagnosis, I contacted Norman Geschwind, the Harvard neurologist who had first publicized the characteristic personalities of TLE patients and who had diagnosed my friend. Over the phone Geschwind referred me to other experts, and we agreed to meet. A week later, the fifty-eight-year-old doctor had a fatal heart attack. In the years that followed, I called the people whose names he had given me, interviewed scores of doctors and patients, observed neurosurgeons performing the surgical treatment for TLE, attended lectures and read articles and books about the disorder, and researched the lives and works of the legion of writers, artists, and religious leaders who are thought by experts to have had TLE.

The stories of these creative luminaries are here interwoven with the stories of three ordinary people: Charlie, an attorney who has had TLE for twenty years; Jill, a corporate executive who developed it ten years ago; and Gloria, a retired hairdresser who has had the disorder nearly all her life. The book recounts medical breakthroughs in the history of TLE, with a focus not only on Geschwind and two earlier physicians who pioneered the modern understanding of the disorder, but also on many other doctors along the way who added pieces to the puzzle. It examines the hidden causes and manifold effects of TLE seizures and the arresting variety of personality traits associated with the disorder, underscoring the similarities and differences between these symptoms and so-called normal behaviors. Finally, the book relates the ways doctors try to intervene in cases of TLE, in both diagnosis and treatment, including the potential misuse of treatment. Throughout the book, these accounts of ordinary and extraordinary experiences with TLE lead to explorations of such abiding human attributes as aggression, sexuality, and creativity, showing the ramifications of this remarkable disorder for all of us.

Seized

CHAPTER ONE

A Classic Case

In 1888, in the south of France, a country doctor made a clever diagnosis. His patient was a thirty-five-year-old Dutch painter who had been living in the village of Arles for ten months. On Christmas morning, police brought the artist to the local hospital, where the doctor, Felix Rey, was on duty. The artist, Rey noted, was delirious, his head bloody; the night before, he had cut off part of his left ear. That afternoon and again the next morning, the two men strolled the hospital grounds, enumerating the patient's troubles over recent months. He had been feeling agitated and depressed. He feared that he was going mad. His brain wasn't working right: he had heard voices, and there were chunks of time that he could not recall. On December 26, the doctor wrote in the patient's hospital chart, "M. van Gogh suffers from a form of epilepsy."

That form of epilepsy, now known as temporal lobe epilepsy, or TLE, consists of seizures in a part of the brain controlling feelings and memories. During a TLE seizure a person is overtaken by a powerful emotion, usually anger or fear, by hallucinatory voices or visions, or by a vivid flashback. The seizure lasts moments or minutes, rarely more than an hour, and it is accompanied by no apparent physical change, except sometimes a dull stare or a trembling of the arm or mouth. During the seizure the person may move about as if sleepwalking and may perform automatic acts, sometimes violent, which she is later unable to recall. Unlike the far better known seizures of grand mal epilepsy, which consists of noticeable bodily convulsions, TLE seizures are not easily recognized. They affect only part—not all—of the brain, and they involve only alteration—not cessation—of consciousness. TLE has been alluded to since the fifth century B.C., when Hippocrates published *The Sacred Disease,* his treatise on the epilepsies. Its designation as a separate disorder, however, is not universally accepted even now: some doctors refuse to say a patient has epilepsy unless he loses consciousness. Despite this diagnostic problem, TLE seizures are today the most common form of seizures in adults: for every two adults with grand mal epilepsy, there are three with TLE.

In van Gogh's time, this form of epilepsy was hardly known. Yet Felix Rey had already seen another patient who sliced off an earlobe and was diagnosed as epileptic. Spurred by a medical-school classmate who had just completed a thesis on the disorder, the young doctor had then read contemporary journal articles on the subject, including those by John Hughlings Jackson, an English neurologist who was one of the first to define TLE. Jackson wrote that there was no objective test for "psychic epilepsy," as he called it, and that only by taking a patient's history could a doctor discover its presence. Using this method, similar to the one still used today in diagnosing TLE, Rey listened to van Gogh and pieced together a picture of how his epilepsy had evolved.

The artist's difficult birth, in 1853 in the village of Zundert in the Netherlands, was at the root of his problem, the doctor suspected. Seizures result from electrical, chemical, or physical problems in the brain; in van Gogh, Rey thought, the cause was physical. Van Gogh's mother's labor had been long, and in the birth canal the baby had briefly been without oxygen. The doctor theorized that a cluster of Vincent's brain cells, starved for oxygen, had been damaged, leaving a little scar, a spot where, years later, seizures could start. Rey noted the striking asymmetry of van Gogh's face, a visible sign of damage to one side of the brain that is consistent with scarring of one hemisphere, which can inhibit the development of one side of the body. Another factor strengthening the diagnosis of epilepsy was the artist's family history of brain disorders: one of his sisters spent her adulthood in a hospital for the insane; his mother's sister had grand mal seizures; and other relatives were diagnosed as epileptic. Rey knew that although epilepsy is not inherited directly, a predisposition to it runs in families.

The artist's early development also signaled to the doctor that something within van Gogh was unusual. Since childhood, van Gogh recalled, he had suffered from periodic headaches, stomach aches, dizziness, and depression. He shunned people, spending most of his time alone. As a young man, hoping to follow his father into the Protestant ministry, he became a missionary, traveling to impoverished Belgian villages to preach Christianity. Though he lacked the necessary stability, his fervor was legendary. He punished himself by refusing to eat and wearing rags. Villagers nicknamed him "God's madman," and church officials dismissed him from one post for his "excess of zeal bordering on the scandalous." In his late twenties, after ten lonely years of evangelical work, he abandoned religion in favor of art. Unable to make a living in either field, he told the doctor, he was supported financially by his father and his younger brother, Theo.

In his early thirties, van Gogh continued, his behavior had become more erratic. He had mystical visions, including one of a resurrected Christ, and frequent attacks of rage. In 1886, overcome by fury in a crowded Paris art gallery, he actually took off all his clothes. This experience reminded Rey of an article he had read about TLE by Jackson: "Probably . . . in cases in which a man all at once passes into a violent rage from no apparent cause, or into a state somewhat like somnambulism, in which he may walk a mile or two, or walk into a canal, or in which he takes off his boots in church, or undresses himself in the streets, there is epilepsy."

About two years after disrobing in the gallery, van Gogh had moved to Arles to paint in the region's beautiful light. Over the next few months he wrote numerous letters to his friend the painter Paul Gauguin, begging him to come to Arles. In October 1888, Gauguin at last arrived and moved into the yellow house that van Gogh had rented and furnished.

Their shared life was easy at first. They spent the days painting and the evenings drinking and talking in cafés. Van Gogh was delighted that Gauguin liked to shop, while he preferred to cook; this simplified their division of chores.

In the past few weeks, van Gogh told Rey, life had suddenly grown hard. He developed terrible stomach pains, lost his appetite, and experienced hallucinations. One day, as he was painting peonies, the right half of his visual field went dark, while the flowers in the left half turned upside down. He became moody and irritable. One December afternoon, as Gauguin completed a portrait of van Gogh at his easel painting sunflowers, van Gogh said of the likeness, "That's me all right, but me gone mad." Increasingly he resented the hours that Gauguin spent with local women and prostitutes. On December 23, as the two men were drinking together in a café, van Gogh suddenly reached for his glass, which contained the cloudy green spirit absinthe, and threw it at Gauguin's head. Gauguin dodged the glass, grabbed van Gogh, and dragged him home to bed.

The next morning, when van Gogh awoke from an unusually deep sleep, Gauguin announced that he would soon leave Arles. Van Gogh pleaded with his friend to stay and apologized profusely for his outburst, which, he admitted, he could hardly recall. Gauguin refused to reconsider. All day he kept his distance. At dusk, he left the house for a walk to the public garden, leaving van Gogh at home alone.

Going to his mirror and taking up his razor, van Gogh began to shave the edges of his ruddy beard. Just then, he told the doctor, he heard a disembodied voice commanding him to kill Gauguin. In Rey's opinion, van Gogh had seized; the voice was a TLE seizure, coming from inside his brain.

Prompted by the voice, van Gogh went out into the empty street. He approached the public garden, passed between the firs and bougainvillea bushes that marked its entrance, and walked along the garden path, the blade still in his hand.

In a few minutes he reached Gauguin who, hearing footsteps, turned to find his host, fifteen feet behind him, looking crazed and holding up a blade. Van Gogh appeared to be in a trance. Moments later, he swung around and ran home, where he used the blade on himself, slicing off the lower half of his ear, the source of the voice that had told him to kill Gauguin.

To stanch the blood gushing from the wound, van Gogh pressed towel after towel to his head, dropping the soiled ones to the floor. Hours passed. Gauguin did not return; he had decided to spend the night at a hotel.

Around midnight, van Gogh picked up his severed ear, wrapped it in paper, and went out. He walked through the village to a brothel that Gauguin frequented, where he left his ear on the stoop with a note saying it was a "keepsake" for a prostitute who had once posed for him. He returned home, escorted by a neighbor who had been alerted to his strange behavior, and went to sleep. The next morning, roused by officers summoned by the neighbor, he was taken to the hospital, where he met Felix Rey.

To treat the condition he diagnosed, Rey prescribed most everything then available for any form of epilepsy. Potassium bromide, a drug first used as an antiepileptic in 1857 and now discontinued, seemed to van Gogh to lessen his "unbearable hallucinations," but otherwise it did not help him. Rey advised the artist to stop drinking alcohol, which in sufficient quantities can cause seizures. Van Gogh had not drunk regularly until 1886, in Paris, when he joined a café-going group of artists, among them Gauguin, Pissarro, and Toulouse-Lautrec. The crowd's favorite spirit, absinthe, is so epileptogenic that it was banned for human use in 1914 and has since been used experimentally to create seizures in dogs. Van Gogh had drunk no absinthe from the time of his departure from Paris, early in 1888, until the recent weeks with Gauguin. Now, when he again stopped drinking and started eating regularly at the hospital, his condition improved.

Two weeks after his admission, van Gogh felt well enough to paint. In fact his desire to work was huge. Among the numerous paintings he did while under Rey's care are a portrait of the doctor and a series of self-portraits with his head bandaged. He also wrote obsessively. Instead of sending his brother Theo one letter a day, as he had before, he now sent two or three letters daily, many of them six or more pages long. By the middle of January, he felt well enough to return to his house.

At the end of the month, however, his seizures returned, and now they were worse. "The storm within," as he called his typical seizure, consisted of hallucinations, unprovoked feelings of anger, confusion, and fear, and floods of early memories that disturbed him because they were outside his control. In one such seizure, he "saw again every room at the house in Zundert" where he had been born, "every path, every plant in the garden, the views in the fields roundabout . . . down to a magpie's nest in a tall acacia in the graveyard." During many seizures, he forgot where he was, or else his surroundings seemed unreal. At times his hearing and vision were affected: nearby voices seemed to come from afar; objects appeared to shrink; and faces were distorted. He suffered "moods of indescribable mental anguish" and an "undercurrent of vague sadness." He became paranoid, suspecting people in the village of wanting to poison him. Early in February, he was readmitted to the hospital, where he threatened Rey with a razor, as he had once threatened Gauguin.

Thus began a pattern that would endure for the rest of van Gogh's short life. From then on, he alternated between periods of near madness and highly productive calm. In the nineteen months that began in December 1888, he required almost constant hospitalization; yet he painted more often and more expressively than ever before, producing hundreds of watercolors, oil paintings, and drawings—nearly half his lifetime output. As he deteriorated in body and mind, he created the canvases for which he is best known, including some of the most coveted works in the history of art.

As he saw it, whatever was destroying him also fueled his painting. He felt himself developing an "excessive sensitivity" to the visual world that he had not known before. "The cypress [I am painting] is always occupying my thoughts," he wrote to Theo from Arles. "It is as beautiful in line and proportion as an Egyptian obelisk, and the green has a quality of high distinction. It is a splash of *black* in a sunny landscape, but it is one of the most interesting of the black notes, and the most difficult to strike exactly that I can imagine. But then you must see the cypress against the blue, *in* the blue rather. To paint nature here, as everywhere, you must have lived in it a long time. I should like to make something of the cypresses like the canvases of the sunflowers; it astonishes me that they have never been done as I see them. . . . Sometimes I draw sketches almost against my will. Is it not emotion, the sincerity of one's feeling for nature, that draws us? And if the emotions are sometimes so strong that one works without knowing one works, when sometimes the strokes come with a continuity and coherence like words in a speech or a letter. . . . One must strike while the iron is hot."

Rey had read in Jackson's writings of a link between "psychic *epilepsy you with anxiety*

epilepsy" and creativity, but he was more concerned about his patient's health than his art, so he ordered van Gogh to rest—not to paint. Van Gogh responded by moving, in May 1889, from the hospital in Arles to an asylum for epileptics and the insane in nearby Saint-Rémy-de-Provence, where he committed himself. The doctor at Saint-Rémy, Theophile-Zacharie-Auguste Peyron, concurred with Rey's diagnosis of epilepsy and his recommendation that van Gogh avoid "mental work." But Peyron offered the artist two cells, one to sleep in and the other in which he could paint.

Van Gogh continued to suffer and produce. In his seizures, which were now "abominable, horrible, terrible," he screamed and cursed, sleepwalked, and undressed in public. One day, while painting in a quarry near the asylum and attended by a hospital worker, van Gogh had a seizure in which his entire body convulsed. "There is quite definitely something or other deranged in my brain," he wrote to his brother. Still, whenever he felt well he worked "like a steam engine," according to his doctor's son. Explaining his motivation to paint in a letter to Theo, Vincent wrote, "Work distracts me, and I *must* have some distraction; or rather work keeps me in control, so that I don't deny myself it . . . I *miss* the work more than it tires me." He added by way of understatement, "I love to paint, The more ugly, old, ill, and poor I get, the more I want to take my revenge by painting in brilliant colors, well-arranged, resplendent."

The desire to express himself artistically was not the only emotion that intensified. His anger and his dependence both were pushed to new extremes. His attacks of rage exploded regularly in threats, insults, and violence toward other patients and his doctors. At Saint-Rémy he twice attempted suicide by swallowing kerosene, oil paint, and turpentine.

His reliance on his brother and on Gauguin also increased. He called his relationship with Theo a "lawful union," as if it were a marriage. Though younger by four years, Theo had at twenty-three assumed the burden of supporting Vincent, sending him money, canvases, and paints, and trying in vain to sell his paintings. The brothers had lived together in Paris from 1886 until early 1888, when Vincent moved to Arles. When Theo became engaged in December 1888, Vincent's happiness for his brother was obscured by his sadness for himself. Feeling abandoned, he desperately tried to transfer his dependency from Theo to Gauguin, who did not play a supporting role nearly as well as Theo. After Vincent cut his ear, for instance, Gauguin left Arles without a word to him, while Theo immediately halted a vacation with his fiancée to nurse his brother. Even so, Vincent had a hard time parting with Gauguin. He continued fantasizing that they would live together again. As late as 1890, he sent Gauguin gifts of paintings and considered following him to Madagascar.

After a year at Saint-Rémy and against his doctor's orders, van Gogh decided to move. Depressed and afraid, he wanted to be near his brother, who now lived in Paris with his wife and infant son. In May 1890, the artist traveled north to the village of Auvers-sur-Oise, where he settled in an inn. From there he visited Theo in Paris, but family obligations prevented Theo from giving his brother the attention he wanted. When Theo decided that to save money he would take his summer holiday at his wife's home in Holland, rather than with Vincent in Auvers, the artist left Paris for Auvers in a rage. A new series of seizures overtook him. He saw horrifying visions, and heard voices. No longer able to work, he fell into despair. On Sunday, July 27, in the afternoon, he walked into a field of hay and shot himself in the chest.

At dusk, he stumbled into the inn where he was staying. Doctors could not remove the bullet. In his coat pocket they found a letter addressed to his brother. "Once back here I set to work again, though the brush almost slipped from my fingers," it read. "Knowing exactly what I wanted, I painted three more big canvases. They are vast stretches of corn under troubled skies, and I did not need to go out of my way to express sadness and extreme loneliness."

Theo, alerted by the doctors, arrived the next day. He found Vincent conscious but near death. Early Tuesday morning, the thirty-seven-year-old painter died in his brother's arms.

In the decades to follow, the diagnosis made by Rey and confirmed by Peyron was largely ignored. To scholars of art, van Gogh's symptoms, except the isolated instance of bodily convulsions in the quarry near Saint-Rémy, sounded nothing like epilepsy. The artist's crises, hospitalizations, and violence instead indicated that he was "crazy," that in him creative genius had somehow coexisted with madness. Psychiatrists, noting his many symptoms that also occur in schizophrenia—incorporeal voices, visions, paranoia, rage, and flights from reality—theorized that he suffered from that mental illness in the last two years of his life. Schizophrenia soon became the strongest competitor in the quest to fix a diagnosis on van Gogh, although neurologists cautioned that his powerful artistic concentration, which persisted until his final days, was inconsistent with the mental deterioration that usually accompanies schizophrenia. Over the years doctors suggested more than a hundred alternative diagnoses—such as syphilis, manic-depressive illness, sunstroke, Ménière's disease, acute intermittent porphyria, glaucoma, and chemical poisoning—each of which was trumpeted in medical journals and just as loudly disavowed.

In the meantime, epilepsy specialists quietly continued to view van Gogh's initial diagnosis as correct. The more neurologists learned about TLE, in fact, the more they found in van Gogh a classic case.

First, his heredity and environment put him at risk for epilepsy. Sixty-five years after his death, a French neurologist named Henri Gastaut studied van Gogh's life and medical records and concluded that his family history implied an inherited susceptibility to the disorder; his facial asymmetry indicated brain damage; and his physical and emotional problems in childhood suggested brain scarring early on, either from a childhood virus, from a long-forgotten fall on the head, or, as Rey had suspected, from birth. While these factors were necessary conditions for seizures, Gastaut added, van Gogh's incipient alcohol use in 1886 set them in motion, causing minor seizures in 1887 and major ones in 1888, which culminated in the violent Christmastime attack. People with undiagnosed TLE sometimes drink alcohol in an attempt to mute the effects of their seizures, unknowingly making them worse. Without alcohol, Gastaut thought, van Gogh's inherent tendency to epilepsy might not have developed into actual seizures.

As it was, the painter did drink and numerous seizure states occurred. Gastaut asserted, "It seems impossible to refute that van Gogh had seizures during the last two years of his life." All of the artist's discrete complaints—from the epigastric distress to the recurrent hallucinations, fear, anger, and seemingly unmotivated outbursts—were consistent with TLE. His many periods without these symptoms, during which he worked furiously, also fit this diagnostic picture, because the frequency of seizures can change from month to month or week to week, as a result of hormonal cycles, rest, and stress, all of which affect brain activity.

Finally, the artist displayed the set of personality traits that neurologists consider a hallmark of TLE. "Van Gogh's personality problems were no different from the character troubles between seizures that are habitually found in people with TLE," Gastaut observed, citing the artist's explosive temper, his extreme dependence on other people, his lack of interest in sex, his "morbid hyperreligiosity," and his compulsion to write and draw. Gastaut noted that these characteristics, in tandem with undiagnosed TLE seizures, were sometimes misdiagnosed as symptoms of psychiatric disease, an error that may have been made posthumously in the case of van Gogh. These characteristics, evident in the painter throughout his life, peaked with his most troubling seizures and with his greatest art. Though wary of "reducing one of the greatest expressions of universal art to psychological considerations," Gastaut nevertheless concluded that through these traits van Gogh's disorder contributed to his work: "The waxing and waning of his character troubles, which resulted from the activation and deactivation of his seizures, must have influenced the evolution of his art and the many variations in his manner of painting as it reached its pinnacle in the south of France."

CHAPTER TWO

Pioneers

For the last thirty-five years of his life, John Hughlings Jackson dined alone at home in London, at a table set for two. The empty place setting was for his wife, Elizabeth Dade Jackson, a writer of children's stories who had died of a stroke before her fortieth birthday. Hughlings, as he was known, and Elizabeth were cousins who had courted for eleven years, from their teens, and wed in 1865. After her death in 1876, he confided to a friend, "There is nothing in the world to compare with domestic happiness." The shy, retiring doctor never married again.

Elizabeth Jackson's fatal stroke was caused by a chronic congenital condition that narrowed the blood vessels to her brain and brought on other problems as well. From time to time she felt as though insects were crawling beneath her skin, a tremor traveled up one side of her body, and she lapsed into a "dreamy state" of several minutes in which objects around her seemed remote or not quite real. These attacks are now easily identified as TLE seizures, but then they were poorly understood. Since the time of ancient Greece, epilepsy has been known as the "falling sickness," a definition that made TLE seizures, most of which do not involve falling down, difficult to identify. Even when TLE seizures were correctly diagnosed as epilepsy, the diagnosis itself was considered a mark of shame. For thousands of years people shunned epileptics, thinking them possessed, their seizures the result of gods or demons inhabiting their heads. In the nineteenth century this view began to fall from favor, but the new consensus among lay people and some doctors was that seizures resulted from sexual excesses or masturbation. As it happened, Elizabeth Jackson's husband was one of the few people alive who knew what epilepsy actually is, where it originates, and why it occurs. Having realized its power to illuminate the brain and the mind, he had devoted himself to understanding the disorder.

Born in 1835, in rural Yorkshire, Hughlings Jackson apprenticed to a doctor in his youth, attended York Medical School, and spent forty-four years as a physician to neurological patients at the renowned National Hospital for the Relief and Cure of the Paralysed and Epileptic, in Queen Square, London. As a clinician he was assiduous, noting "exactly what the patient did and said, his every delay, hesitancy, faulty response, and gesture," his younger colleague Macdonald Critchley reported. "This was only the beginning. He went on to ponder, and to ask himself—why? He strove to unravel the fundamental problems which pervaded the nervous system and which resulted in that particular pattern of altered function." In the process Jackson recorded scores of his patients' seizure states, among them hallucinatory smells and tastes, the momentary inability to move a limb or to understand words, and the odd sensations, tremors, and dreamy states that his wife had experienced. His study of many patients continued beyond their deaths, when he dissected their brains at autopsy and wrote detailed case histories of what he had found.

Away from his work, the doctor was withdrawn and absent-minded. On the day he was supposed to show Queen Victoria around the wards of the National Hospital, for instance, he forgot to arrive. Social and cultural affairs bored him, with one exception: he loved to read, especially the novels of Austen and Dickens and popular thrillers by William Wilkie Collins and Arthur Conan Doyle. But books themselves meant nothing to Jackson. He often tore out and discarded pages as he read them, and even cut from borrowed neurology texts the sections he wanted to reread. One afternoon, a salesboy in a bookstore gawked as the prim, bearded doctor tore off the cover of a volume he had just purchased and ripped the text in two, so as to fit half the book in each coat pocket. Catching the boy's stare, Jackson solemnly explained, "You think I'm mad, my boy, but it's the people who don't do this who are mad."

Jackson's neurological interests were vast, encompassing movement disorders, speech disorders, and "insanities," but epilepsy was the disorder about which he wrote the most. In a series of articles that began in 1861 with "Cases of Epilepsy Associated with Syphilis" and ended in 1902 with "Observations on a Case of Convulsions," he laid the foundation for the modern view of epilepsy.

His conception of the disorder rested on his early identification of what a seizure is. In 1862, when the young doctor arrived at the National Hospital, researchers had already begun to suspect that seizures are organic, the result of an undetermined physical problem in the brain. One theory, which initially impressed Jackson, held that seizures are the brain's response to poisons in the blood. Jackson modified this idea, suggesting that seizures occur when blood vessels to the brain contract, "diminishing the quantity of the blood." This appeared to explain the seizures of his wife and other patients with vascular disorders, but it did not explain the seizures of the many epileptic patients who displayed no evidence of reduced blood supply to the brain. Jackson knew there had to be another factor underlying seizures, which every epileptic shared.

That factor was a scar. Without exception, the brains of epileptic patients on whom Jackson performed autopsies contained visibly damaged tissue. These scars had a variety of causes—such as head injuries, alcohol or chemical poisoning, the pressure of growing tumors, or the temporary loss of oxygen or blood—but it was the scar, rather than any single cause, that correlated with seizure states.

Jackson knew that the brain is composed of nerve cells that contribute to human actions, feelings, and thoughts by "firing," or producing electrical charges. He theorized that the cells in or around a scar, unable to fire normally because they are damaged, occasionally produce "discharges," or uncontrolled bursts of electricity, and that whenever this happens, a seizure occurs. In 1873 he wrote, "Epilepsy is the name for occasional, sudden, excess, rapid and local discharges of grey matter," or brain tissue. This definition, now famous, is surprisingly terse, given that elsewhere he required eleven pages to define the disorder. He later proposed a jocular metaphor for epileptic brain cells: they are a "mad part" of the brain that makes nearby "sane cells . . . act madly."

The realization that epilepsy consists of misfiring electricity in the brain enabled Jackson to construct an all-encompassing theory of seizures and seizure disorders. The word *epilepsy*, from the Greek *epilēpsia*, meaning to take, or seize, as if from outside, refers to any disorder consisting of recurring seizure states. Unlike his contemporaries, who believed that only grand mal seizures constitute "true" or "genuine" epilepsy, Jackson discerned at least two "epilepsies," which are distinguished by the extent of the misfiring. In grand mal seizures, he observed, the epileptic discharge rapidly spreads across the brain, producing a kind of vast, internal electrical storm that shuts down higher functions and causes the person to lose consciousness, fall down, and experience bodily convulsions; Jackson called these seizures "generalized." In the second category of seizures, the spread of the epileptic activity remains within a limited region of the brain; these seizures he called "localized," or "focal."

Jackson's distinction persists: today doctors refer to seizures as either "generalized" or "partial," the latter category including TLE. Generalized seizures include both grand mal seizures and petit mal, or absence, seizures, in which awareness lapses momentarily. Partial seizures are either simple or complex, depending on whether consciousness is altered. Not all complex partial seizures are specifically TLE, but many doctors now use the terms "complex partial seizure disorder" and TLE interchangeably. While the two broad categories of seizure are distinct, a partial seizure can "generalize," progressing within minutes into a grand mal attack. A person whose TLE seizures regularly generalize is said to have "secondary generalized partial seizures."

Partial seizures commanded the bulk of Jackson's attention because they appeared to provide a window into the functions of selected regions of the brain. The function of the region where the discharge occurs determines the content of the seizure state, because the discharge interferes with this particular function, temporarily turning it on or off. Epileptic discharge in a brain region involved in the sensation of smell, for instance, can cause seizures in which a person either hallucinates a smell or is temporarily unable to smell anything. Epileptic discharge in Jackson's wife altered several ordinary functions: movement, when her limbs trembled; sensation, when her skin crawled; and consciousness or memory, during her dreamy states. While Jackson naturally did not perform an autopsy on his own wife, he noted at numerous other autopsies that epileptic brain scars were usually located in a region thought to control the function that had been affected at the beginning of the patient's typical seizure state. This confirmed his view that the location of the discharge correlated with the seizure's effects.

These theories are widely accepted today, and their progenitor is known as the father of modern neurology, but they were at first "passed over in contemptuous silence," the physician Henry Head observed in 1911. Jackson lacked the skill or the desire to promote his work: a weak lecturer who despised traveling, he avoided the medical conferences at which doctors gather to exchange ideas. Moreover, there was resistance in Victorian England to ascribing dreamy states, hallucinations, and disrobing in public to anything other than moral or sexual flaws. In fact, English doctors overlooked Jackson's findings until doctors on the Continent, who had read his articles in French and German translations, alerted them to read him in the original. One of these European doctors was Felix Rey; another was Sigmund Freud, the father of psychiatry, who in the 1880s began his career as a neurologist, examining the nerve cells of crayfish, eels, and human fetuses. One more reason why Jackson's contributions to epilepsy were initially overlooked is that they were based on ideas that were not yet proven. Jackson was not an experimenter, but a theorist; his ideas arose from his observations of patients and from his powers of intuition. "The use of hypothesis," he explained, "is the method of science. . . . An hypothesis, otherwise a supposition, is not a conclusion. It is only the starting point for methodical observation and experiment."

As experimenters began to verify his hypotheses, Jackson's

reputation grew. In the 1870s, German scientists named Fritsch and Hitzig made a dog's limbs move by sending weak currents into tissues near the front of its exposed brain, demonstrating that electrical currents to the brain cause involuntary movements. Lengthening the period of stimulation or increasing the current caused the dog to have a generalized convulsion. Almost simultaneously, in England, Richard Caton used a wire and a voltage meter to demonstrate in rabbits and cats the natural "electric currents in the brain." And Jackson's Scottish colleague Sir David Ferrier created artificial epilepsy in monkeys by sending electric currents down wires implanted in their brains. Stimulated in one spot, Ferrier's monkeys had tremors; in another spot, they bared their teeth and growled; in a third spot, they cowered. These diverse reactions to stimulation of different parts of the brain suggested that functions are "localized" in certain brain regions. This provided an explanation for Jackson's theory that epileptic discharge in different brain regions causes different seizural effects. Eventually some monkeys seized without any external charge; Ferrier reasoned that his repeated stimulation of their brains had created a scar able to produce a seizure on its own. When he killed the animals and removed and examined their brains, he was able to see these scars.

But there were limits to the methods available to prove Jackson's ideas. Fritsch and Hitzig, Caton, and Ferrier operated on animal brains because experimentation on the pulsing brains of humans was not allowed. With the exception of rare surgical procedures to remove life-threatening tumors, doctors could observe the live human brain only indirectly—in action, as a person functioned. The brains of live animals could be probed, cut, dyed, altered, and removed, but the brains of live humans could not. Given this ethical constraint, researchers learned what they could about the human brain by experimenting on the brains of rabbits, monkeys, and dogs. The dissimilarities between animal and human brains were left for theorists to ponder and future researchers to explore.

Oscar Wilde could have been describing Jackson when he wrote, "There are some works which wait and which one does not understand for a long time; the reason is that they bring answers to questions that have not yet been raised." The daring of Jackson's thought and the restriction against experimenting on humans prevented his ideas about epilepsy from being fully investigated in his lifetime. In October 1911, when he died of pneumonia at seventy-six and his body was buried beside his wife's in London's Highgate cemetery, no one could be sure that the dreamy states of his wife and his patients were the result, as he thought, of electrical discharges in the brain. For another quarter-century, Jackson's proof would have to wait.

On an operating table in a Montreal surgical theater in the 1930s, a twenty-six-year-old woman lay on her left side. Her head was shaved; a metal frame held it still. The right side of her scalp was pulled back and a piece of her skull had been removed, revealing a four-inch-square patch of her brain. She was fully conscious; a local anesthetic prevented her from feeling anything in her scalp and the tissues covering her brain, but since the organ that creates pain itself feels no pain, general anesthesia was not used.

A charged probe, an insulated wire carrying two volts of electricity, hovered above the wet, knotty surface of her brain. The neurosurgeon who held the probe, Wilder Penfield, had repeatedly touched it to the exposed brain, each time observing her response, which indicated the function of the region he had touched. Penfield knew that in humans, as in Ferrier's monkeys, electrical stimulation of brain tissue activates the function controlled by that tissue: an involuntary movement of the woman's tongue told him that his probe had touched a region involved in movement; when she reported tingling in her thumb, he knew he had found a region controlling sensation; and her momentary inability to speak signaled an area involved in speech. These regions controlling movement, sensation, and speech were of special interest to Penfield, who was about to perform brain surgery in the hope of treating the woman's epilepsy, because they were areas that he wanted to be sure not to remove.

Now, as his probe touched her brain, something unexpected occurred. "I heard something," the woman said to Penfield, her voice muffled by the heavy surgical fabric that separated the incision on her scalp from her face. "I don't know what it is." It seemed to her to be a memory.

Full of wonder, Penfield gently returned the probe to the spot it had touched before. "Yes, sir," the woman said. "I think I heard a mother calling her little boy somewhere. It seemed to be something that happened years ago. It was somebody in the neighborhood where I live, and I was close enough to hear."

The touch of the charged wire to her brain had brought to consciousness a moment in her past. The memory was as vivid as though it were a present experience, yet she remained aware of being in an operating room in Montreal. The experience was like a dream in which her mind had split in two, one part in the present, the other part experiencing the moment long ago. This feeling was familiar to the woman; it reminded her of feelings she had had during her partial seizures.

Penfield had seen patients report vivid, seizurelike memories in response to electrical stimulation of the brain only twice before. On the first occasion, in 1933, also prior to surgery for epilepsy, he had been "incredulous," thinking the reaction an exception or a coincidence. Now, realizing that he might be on the verge of discovering the nature of Jackson's dreamy state, Penfield "marvelled" at what he had found.

Keeping his excitement to himself, he quietly informed the patient that he was about to stimulate her again. His hand, invisible to her, descended toward a new spot nearby, and the probe touched down on her brain. "Yes," she said, indicating that she had had another memory. "I heard voices down along the river—a man's voice and a woman's voice calling. . . . I think I saw the river." The second memory evoked by the probe was seen as well as heard.

Continuing backward, the probe delicately landed again. This time the woman reported a *déjà vu* experience—"a tiny flash of familiarity"—and also "the feeling that I knew everything that was going to happen in the near future." Probed in a slightly different spot, she cried, "Oh!" and described another "very familiar memory," of being in an office whose location she could not place. "I could see the desks, and someone was calling to me, a man leaning on a desk with a pencil in his hand." With the wire to her brain, her mind's eye saw the man. The moment the wire moved away, he disappeared.

Penfield was almost certain that these memories were simulations of the seizures that Jackson had called dreamy states. To verify that the woman's response was the result of electricity rather than of suggestion, he moved his hand slightly and warned her that he was about to stimulate her, but he kept the probe from touching her brain. "Nothing," she said. Silently he stimulated another spot not far from the others. "I had a little memory," she reported, "a scene in a play. They were talking and I could see it. I was just seeing it in my memory."

It was now clear to the surgeon that these memories resulted directly from the application of electrical charges to one region of the brain—the same region, he thought, that must be activated during dreamy states. He had "stumbled," Penfield said later, "upon the fact that electrical stimulation of the interpretive areas of the cortex"—brain regions devoted to memory and perception "occasionally produces what Hughlings Jackson had called 'dreamy states.'" Almost by accident, a surgeon had proven what a theorist had conceived.

The surgeon had been born in Spokane, Washington, in 1891, the son of a frontier doctor and a genteel Christian Scientist. His parents separated for good when Penfield was eight, his mother returning with the children to her family home in Wisconsin. Penfield attended Princeton University, where he won a Rhodes scholarship. He studied neurology in the United States and Europe, spending a year in London at the Queen Square hospital with Jackson's former students and colleagues. While working as a field doctor in France during the First World War, he was attracted to surgery, which he observed to be "nothing but skilled carpentry work with a lot of daring, knowledge of anatomy and pathology and judgement. I'm glad I've done some carpentering—the rest must be hammered out." He began his career as a neurosurgeon in 1921, in New York City. Seven years later he moved with his wife and children to Montreal, where McGill University and the Royal Victoria Hospital had invited him to start an institute devoted to neurology. Only the second neurosurgeon to work full time in Canada, Penfield remained there until his death in 1976.

Like Jackson, Penfield had epilepsy in his family. From childhood his older sister, Ruth, had suffered from brief alterations in consciousness that were not recognized as partial seizures. These attacks worsened in her forties to include grand mal seizures that demanded medical attention. With an ophthalmoscope, an instrument championed by Jackson, Penfield looked at the back of his sister's eyes, where swollen veins and optic nerves suggested the presence of a brain tumor. The tumor, which was thought to have been present since child-hood, caused seizures by pressing on healthy brain tissue; as it expanded from inside her brain toward her face, the kind of seizure she experienced had changed from partial to grand mal. Penfield, one of the few doctors in the world equipped to remove the tumor, decided to perform the chancy operation himself. This display of brotherly resolve was all the more remarkable in light of Ruth's faith in Christian Science, and it offered proof of Penfield's statement that "the only certain virtue that came into the world with me was tenacity of pur-pose. Some would say this is stubbornness."

During the operation on his sister, Penfield found that the tumor had penetrated crucial brain areas, forcing him to leave some of it behind. Over the next eighteen months Ruth's seizures continued, the tumor regrew, and her personality disintegrated so that she could no longer even prepare a simple meal. A sur-geon in Boston removed more tumor. Ruth had a brief period of recovery, but her seizures returned, and she died of the tumor within a year.

Ruth's two conditions—brain tumor and epilepsy—were Pen-field's surgical specialties. Operations on brain tumors gave sur-geons the opportunity to examine the living human brain directly. But brain tumors were rare and often fatal, and the out-come of operations to remove them was frequently poor. Epi-lepsy offered surgeons the same opportunity to explore the working brain, and it had none of the disadvantages of brain tumors; it was prevalent, and neither it nor the operation to treat it, which involved removal of the region where seizures were thought to start, customarily led to a patient's death. Moreover, as Penfield realized in the 1930s while provoking the twenty-six-year-old woman's dreamy states, epilepsy could be produced artificially. With a charged probe during a brain operation, a sur-geon could now create "a reasonable facsimile of the experi-ments nature so frequently performs, with obscure methods, in epileptic patients."

Penfield replicated these "experiments nature so frequently performs" in more than a thousand patients with seizures, never once violating the longstanding prohibition against experimenting on live humans. Since his purpose in surgery was to treat a disorder, in probing the brain he broke no rule. Once inside a patient's brain to treat epilepsy, he could explore the normal workings of the organ. In most cases, he knew, the only difference between an epileptic brain and a normal brain is a "seizure focus," the tiny scar where seizures start. If surgeons probed a normal brain with charged wires, it, too, would "seize."

By making normal parts of the brain accessible to this limited experimentation, epilepsy satisfied Penfield's dual professional aims—to treat neurological disorders, and to understand the brain. "Opportunity-to-learn walks into the operating room with any surgeon who has unanswered questions in his mind," Penfield explained. "Opportunity stands at his elbow . . . as he works on the exposed brain. . . . Like an unseen Puck, it whispers to him . . . : 'This chance may never come again. Stop for just a moment. Consider. Apply the electrode. Listen to what the patient says. Control and verify his response critically while you still can.'" The words Penfield chose to have inscribed on a stone slab outside the door of the Montreal Neurological Institute at its opening in 1934 also described him: "Dedicated to Relief of Sickness and Pain and to the Study of Neurology." Years later he acknowledged the link between these two aims when he wrote that the institute had given him, "at last, facilities for studying the human brain as well as for treating its disabilities," to which he added, "Our purpose, of course, was always to cure."

The operation that he hoped would cure epilepsy was a lobectomy, in which a surgeon uses a scalpel, a suction device, or a noose of silk thread to remove some or all of the lobe of the brain containing the seizure focus. This is usually the temporal lobe, the brain region most likely to develop seizures, for which TLE is named. Emotion and memory, the functions controlled by the temporal lobe, are reflected in TLE seizures, which include dreamy states. Henri Gastaut thought that the alterations of emotion and memory in van Gogh's seizures—panic, rage, fear, flashbacks, and amnesia—indicated that the painter's epileptic scar was in this part of his brain. Van Gogh himself was still alive when the first temporal lobectomies were performed. At one of the earliest, in London in 1886, Hughlings Jackson and

Sir David Ferrier were observers in the operating room. As the surgeon closed the head of the patient, a young Scot whose seizures had developed after a fall from a horse, Jackson commented wryly to Ferrier, who was himself a Scot, "Awful, perfectly awful. . . . We had the chance of getting a joke into the head of a Scotsman and we failed to take advantage of it." In its fifty-year history prior to Penfield, the temporal lobectomy had met with mixed success. Some patients had no seizures or fewer seizures than before, but many patients recovered to find that their seizures were unchanged and that some essential function, such as movement, speech, or memory, was impaired. These losses occurred because surgeons, unable to pinpoint the location in the brain of either the seizure focus or normal functions, accidentally removed regions controlling functions and left the seizure focus behind.

Luckily for Penfield's patients, a recent invention had improved doctors' ability to detect seizure focuses and the functions that a brain region controls. In Germany in 1929, as Penfield was setting up his institute in Montreal, a psychiatrist named Hans Berger had designed a device to measure the electrical currents of the brain. This device, an electroencephalograph, consists of a box emanating eight or sixteen insulated wires with silver electrodes at their tips. Each electrode is placed at a different spot on a person's scalp or brain, and its wire transmits the electrical activity from that area to the box, where a contraption of pens over a moving scroll of paper produces a graph of the brain activity. The result is an electroencephalogram, or EEG, a page of eight or sixteen wavy tracings. Each tracing provides a record of what is happening in one region of the brain. Alterations in the height and width of the waves indicate the activation of ordinary functions such as movement and sensation. Light sleep, deep sleep, calm, excitement, and damaged tissue all display unique EEG patterns, as does death, when the EEG flattens to a line. Seizures, which are intermittent events, and seizure focuses, which are continually present in the brain, have several EEG trademarks. The most reliable sign of a seizure focus is a series of rhythmic "spikes" resulting from rapid, synchronous changes in electrical potential, which sometimes alternate with smoother, lower-voltage waves, producing a "spike-and-wave." Seizures appear on the EEG as jagged, bounc-

ing lines, which electroencephalographers call hypersynchronous action. With these indexes of normal and abnormal activity, a surgeon stimulating a patient's brain before an operation
now had, in addition to the patient's physical or verbal response,
an objective measure of the amount and location of electrical
changes in the brain.

In the early 1930s, Penfield acquired an EEG machine and
hired the electroencephalographer Herbert Jasper, one of a new
breed of doctors expert in reading the EEG. Jasper commuted
weekly between a hospital in Rhode Island and Penfield's institute in Canada, carrying the EEG machine in the backseat of his
car, until 1937, when Penfield lured him to Montreal full time.
Over three decades the two doctors collaborated in stimulating
the brains of hundreds of epileptic patients before and after
lobectomies, initially finding the seizure focus and determining
which functional tissues not to remove, and later verifying that
essential functions were still intact. In the operating room, Penfield would stand, charged probe in hand, by the patient's head,
while Jasper sat above and behind him in a raised glass cubicle
equipped with microphones and the electroencephalograph, its
snakelike wires culminating in the silver-tipped electrodes that
rested on the brain. Whenever the EEG or the patient's words or
behavior indicated that the probe had stimulated a function,
Penfield placed a small round ticket marked with a number
directly on the spot on the brain that the probe had touched; in
case the ticket was moved or lost during the operation, a photog-
rapher and a secretary perched in an observation gallery
recorded each function as found.

In the course of stimulating the brains of numerous patients,
Penfield and Jasper "mapped," or diagramed, many ordinary
functions, including speech, movement, the five senses, emotion,
and memory. In 1954 they compiled these findings in *Epilepsy
and the Functional Anatomy of the Brain*, a book they dedicated
to Jackson because so many of its conclusions "were long ago
[his] surmise." They called the book "an honest record of the
workings of the human brain in normal and abnormal states,"
defining "normal states" as ordinary mental states, and "abnormal states" as the same experiences in partial seizures. They
excluded generalized seizures from their findings because it is
impossible to determine the location in the brain of the initial

discharge in most generalized seizures, due to the rapid spread of the seizure activity throughout the brain. The doctors' accounts of hundreds of their patients' seizures confirmed Jackson's theory that seizure states reflect the normal function of the area where discharge occurs: visual hallucinations arise from visual areas; fear and rage arise from areas controlling emotion; and dreamy states arise from regions involved in consciousness and memory. "It is clear enough," Penfield wrote, that stimulating a seizure with a probe is "activating a normal mechanism in the brain." Consequently, "each seizure provides a glimpse of a partially separable mechanism within the total function of man's master organ."

A vast number of the seizures uncovered by Penfield and Jasper involved abnormalities of memory. A schoolteacher from New York named Jessie reported that her typical seizure started with a complex *déjà vu*, "a complete sequence of recollective thoughts, such as the following: Morning shall pass, then noon, then we shall have evening; or for instance, this house was built, it shall be destroyed, and another shall be built and it will be destroyed. Haven't these thoughts occurred before?"

Other patients reported that ordinary attempts to remember something prompted a seizure. "For example," Sylvère, a Canadian soldier, told Penfield, "if I thought I had seen you somewhere, perhaps in a crowd, and if I tried to make certain in my mind whether I had seen you or not, I might have an attack." This connection of normal memory with seizures led Penfield to conclude that they involved the same brain mechanism: "When this patient tried to make normal use of that mechanism, he evidently precipitated an epileptogenic discharge."

Some patients experienced unwilled memories in seizures and were amnesic afterward, a phenomenon suggesting to Penfield that epileptic firing can activate a function abnormally and then shut it off. At the start of Sylvère's seizures, for instance, he usually heard a voice repeating his name, which Penfield thought was a memory or a pastiche of remembered words. As the seizure continued, Sylvère felt nauseated, dizzy, and fearful. Then he performed an action mechanically, picking at his shirt or walking aimlessly and mumbling, for half a minute or so, unaware of what he was doing. If someone questioned him later about this activity, he said he had no memory of it. Penfield called this seizure state, in which consciousness and memory are impaired, an "automatism."

Van Gogh had sliced off an ear and removed his clothes during apparent automatisms, and the behavior of Penfield's patients during these states likewise tended toward the bizarre. The mother of a New York teenager named Nancy reported that during extended automatisms her daughter appeared confused, smacked her lips, rubbed her stomach, and asked to go to the toilet. Until Nancy was sixteen, these seizures occurred only at home. Then, at a formal ball, she suddenly unzipped her gown, pushed down her underclothes, and squatted as if to urinate. Her friends crowded around her to conceal what she was doing. Still in a state of altered consciousness and finding her clothes about her ankles, Nancy said, "Well, if they are off, we had better take them off completely." She undressed to the skin and attempted to stuff her underpants, slip, and gown into her handbag. Moments later when her normal consciousness returned, she realized she was naked and was overcome with shame. This seizure prompted her to consult a doctor, who recommended that she consult Penfield and consider a lobectomy, in the hope of ending her seizures.

At the Montreal Neurological Institute, an EEG with scalp electrodes showed abnormal electrical activity coming from the temporal lobe on the right side of Nancy's brain. To Penfield, this was good news. Operations on the left half of the brain risk damage to speech and language comprehension, functions that are usually controlled there, so he discouraged surgical candidates whose seizures began in their left hemisphere.

Left Lang

In the operating room, Penfield opened Nancy's skull over the damaged lobe. No physical abnormality was visible. The surgeon suspected that the lobe contained an unseen scar, caused by a high fever when Nancy was two. While traveling abroad with her parents, the toddler had contracted malaria, which brought on the fever and convulsions; her seizures had started a few months later.

In search of Nancy's seizure focus, Penfield repeatedly touched her temporal lobe with his probe. Stimulation of a spot near the front of the lobe elicited a chewing movement and a dazed look. After Penfield withdrew the probe, Nancy told him that she had felt panic, a nauseating sensation of her abdomen "rising," and a "far-off" feeling, as if objects in the room had shrunk. "That," she said, "was an attack."

Having found the seizure focus, Penfield removed the front half of Nancy's right temporal lobe. While his predecessors had removed as little brain tissue as possible in the hope of preserving functions, Penfield made large removals in order to excise all possible epileptic scars. He knew that healthy brain tissue near epileptic tissue often becomes epileptogenic. When his presurgical stimulations indicated that a patient's damaged tissue overlapped with "indispensable" tissue controlling sensation, movement, or speech, Penfield had to choose between leaving some damaged tissue and risking partial loss of vision, for example, or motor control. Another change he made in the procedure was to leave empty the hole he had made in the brain. Other surgeons filled the space with fat or other tissue, often introducing bacteria, but Penfield guessed correctly that cerebrospinal fluid, which bathes the brain, would safely fill it.

When Nancy recovered from the trauma of the operation, her seizures were gone. The one negative aftereffect was a blind spot in the left upper quadrant of her vision, caused by inadvertent damage during surgery to the right side of her brain, which controls the left side of the body. Two years later, she had a few attacks of dizziness that were thought to be seizures, a problem that soon went away. She never disrobed unintentionally again.

Sylvère was another beneficiary of Penfield's dexterity. Twenty-four years old when he went to the institute for treatment, the soldier had had partial seizures for six years. An EEG showed abnormal electrical activity coming from part of his right temporal lobe. At the time of surgery, the reason was obvious. The lobe was visibly enlarged. Measured with a ruler, it was one centimeter longer than Penfield expected. For unknown reasons, some of the tissue had died, and in its place a cyst had developed, expanding the lobe. Penfield made a "large" removal of eight centimeters, including a good deal of healthy tissue.

Following the removal, Penfield set his stimulator at sixty cycles and one volt, probed his conscious patient's brain, and quickly found that Sylvère's speech, sensation, and movement were all in working order. Increasing the voltage on the stimulator to two, the surgeon explored the remaining tissue of the right temporal lobe, eliciting verbal and musical hallucinations that reminded Sylvère of seizure states. Probed in various spots, Sylvère heard a crowd whispering in his left ear, a male voice uttering unintelligible words, and a woman calling a name. Two spots elicited musical memories: a piano rendition of a song that he could not identify; and someone singing the theme song of the radio show "Life of Luigi." Lying on the operating table, Sylvère voluntarily sang the song's refrain. Probed in another spot, he experienced the most common harbinger of his seizure states: he heard his first name spoken in his left ear. These remnants of seizure states did not indicate to Penfield that some of Sylvère's epileptic tissue remained. Even after removing a patient's seizure focus, Penfield was often able to stimulate the altered states of consciousness that patients had known during seizures, because his probe replaced the seizure focus, activating tissues that had formerly been activated only in seizures. In fact, anyone will seize if stimulated with sufficient electricity in the right place.

As Penfield closed the incision on Sylvère's head, Sylvère had two seizures in which the left side of his face twitched. Since twitching was not a normal feature of his seizures, the doctor concluded that these movements resulted from surgical disturbance of brain activity. An EEG done days later showed that all epileptic discharge was gone; apparently all damaged tissue had been removed. Sylvère left the hospital "in good condition" eighteen days after the operation and never had another seizure.

Not every temporal lobectomy ended so well. One in three of Penfield's surgical patients did not improve. Their seizure focuses intact after the operation because of inaccessibility or uncertain location, these patients continued to seize as often as they had before. Jessie, the teacher whose seizures began with the complex *déjà vu*, had a partial right temporal lobectomy at the institute when she was twenty-six. For six months afterward, she had no seizures. Then they returned in slightly altered form. The original *déjà vu* was replaced by a dreamy state in which she felt she was in a car driven by her father in Fordham Square in New York, an actual childhood memory. In other respects, her new seizures were the same as the old: she briefly stopped breathing, she had a terrifying vision of a menacing figure, her abdomen seemed to "rise," she experienced a powerful thirst and cried out for water, her muscles tensed, her head and eyes rolled to the left, and—as the misfiring in her brain generalized—she lost consciousness. Frustrated by the resurgence of these incapacitating attacks, she returned to the institute, where doctors determined that her epileptic scars were too diffuse to justify another operation.

Whether or not a temporal lobectomy helped a given patient, it helped Penfield by providing him with a window on the mind. The pre- and post-surgical stimulations that he performed on Jessie, Sylvère, Nancy, and hundreds of other patients enabled him to prove Jackson's revolutionary theories: that epilepsy is electrical in nature; that its effects are psychic as well as physical, involving memories and emotions as well as bodily convulsions; and that these effects provide evidence of the location in the brain of normal functions, both psychic and physical. The surgeon came a long way in understanding what happens during seizures, but he left others to explain what happens between seizures.

In 1945, on a battlefield not far from the border of Germany and Czechoslovakia, Norman Geschwind, a nineteen-year-old infantryman from New York City, watched in horror as a fellow soldier jumped up as if he had been ordered to attack, drawing deadly enemy fire. The entire time, his commanding officer had been shouting, "Stay low!" to the troops. Geschwind, a brilliant son of Jewish Polish immigrants, who had already completed two years at Harvard College when he was drafted the year before, had seen other soldiers in combat fail to follow the repeated order to lie low. This behavior intrigued him. Why, he wondered, did logic and instinct clash at moments of extreme stress? What brain activity underlay his comrades' self-destructiveness?

After the war, Geschwind completed his undergraduate and medical studies at Harvard. In the footsteps of Penfield and Jackson, he spent three years as a fellow in neurology at the Queen Square hospital in London, where he met his future wife, a nurse. Returning to Boston, he went on to become a professor at Harvard Medical School and chief of neurology at Boston City Hospital. He gained renown throughout the world for his study of the physical underpinnings of human behavior. In 1972, at grand rounds, a weekly teaching session for doctors, Geschwind, now bald and wearing a goatee, sat at a table in a Boston City Hospital library, fidgeting with his pipe and preparing to discuss the disorder that he thought best demonstrates the links between brain activity and human behavior.

After treating people with a variety of neurological disorders for more than twenty years, he told his medical staff, he was convinced that the brain scars that cause TLE seizures also cause personality change. Patients with TLE, he asserted, share "a tendency to increased and extensive" drawing or "writing often of a cosmic or philosophical nature," even when they are not seizing. He called this tendency "hypergraphia," and he speculated that it results from ongoing overstimulation of temporal-lobe tissues by the abnormal electrical activity generated by an epileptic scar. This overstimulation, he thought, enhances the tissues' normal functions of emotion and memory, causing patients to feel experiences unusually deeply, to imbue those experiences with religious or moral significance, and to record them compulsively in drawing or writing.

To some of those listening, the notion of a direct link between TLE, a physical disorder, and complex behaviors like drawing and writing was extraordinary. Stephen Waxman, for one, didn't believe it. "The idea that a specific behavioral change could have a distinct anatomical basis"—the epileptic scar—struck the twenty-seven-year-old resident in neurology as "one of the most bizarre things I've ever heard." Waxman had seen in the medical literature of the nineteenth century isolated articles linking epilepsy with numerous socially unacceptable traits—selfishness, reclusivity, clinginess, extreme religiosity, volatility, paranoia, malice, and criminality, to name a few—but he had dismissed that concept of an "epileptic personality," like the earlier notion that epileptics are possessed, as the product of ignorance and prejudice. Throughout his training, Waxman had been taught to view physical disorders and personality as separate categories. Cancer and emphysema do not affect personality, he knew, so why should epilepsy? Although he usually respected his supervisor's judgment, in this instance he was sure that Geschwind was wrong. Vaguely hoping to prove his point, Waxman determined to scrutinize his patients with TLE.

Weeks later, a patient surprised him by mentioning during an interview that she recorded her seizures in a daily journal. The young doctor questioned her about the journal, and she offered to show it to him. She brought him several thick volumes, and since he seemed interested, she later brought more volumes. To his amazement, they were cross-referenced and organized by category into headache books, seizure books, and special events books. This patient, at least, exhibited Geschwind's hypergraphia "in spades."

Waxman queried other patients about their writing, and many replied that they, too, wrote a great deal. A young man kept a meticulous, typed record of his life. "It was cool last night so I opened the windows and left the air conditioner off," a typical entry reads. "I hung three pictures today on three 3/4 screws I put in the wall." A woman compulsively made lists—of her records, her furniture, and the words of songs her father could play on the harmonica—and repeatedly sketched the sites of her religious experiences. Another patient showed the doctor extensive written descriptions of all her religious feelings, each line of text in alternating colors, red and blue. Inspecting his patients' writings, Waxman found other graphic quirks, such as mirror writing (words written in reverse so that they appear correctly in a mirror), compulsive underlining, and extensive doodling and drawing in the margins. The topic of the writing often bore no relationship to the patient's work or education: a middle-aged woman who had not completed grade school presented shopping bags full of notations on philosophy and religion. Waxman was "blown away," he said, "to hear inner-city patients who were almost functionally illiterate saying, 'I want to write a novel,' and writing lots of poetry, and presenting reams and reams of their writings on philosophical topics." The style of the writing tended to be digressive, repetitious, and driven. A man who produced a detailed, emotional, fifty-six-page medical autobiography had dictated it for seventeen straight hours to a stenographer "because I couldn't write fast enough." A compulsive writer of songs, poems, and aphorisms (such as "Silence is the greatest art of observing") who also kept a diary, explained, "Once I start writing, I can't stop." Patients were "debilitated," Waxman observed, by their desire to write; "writing was all they could do." The skeptical resident began to wonder whether Geschwind could be right.

Working together now, the two doctors developed a test of the possible link between writing and TLE in a larger group of patients. They sent a letter to all their patients—people with various neurological disorders, among them the epilepsies—asking for written descriptions of their present condition. The results were striking: TLE patients responded far more often than patients with other disorders, including patients with other forms of epilepsy, and many of their letters were unusually long. While less than 25 percent of patients with other kinds of epilepsy responded, more than 50 percent of patients with TLE did so, and their letters contained an average of twelve times more words than the letters of other epileptics. As Waxman said, "You could practically *weigh* the responses and pick out" the people with TLE.

In the meantime, he watched for other "personality features" that Geschwind had mentioned at grand rounds, which were the same group of traits that Gastaut had noted in van Gogh. When Waxman questioned his TLE patients about their religious feelings, "many said they believed they were being controlled from outside, by God or by creatures from outer space." One patient ritually recorded in a ledger every day that he was free of seizures, "I thank 'GOD' no seizures." To Waxman's astonishment, multiple religious conversions were common among these patients. A compulsive mirror-writer reported having had five conversions between the ages of seventeen and twenty-one. A man who developed TLE in his thirties abruptly became interested in religion, volunteering daily for religious organizations and determining to become a minister. His sermons dealt with moral issues in "highly circumstantial and meticulous detail." Geschwind had emphasized that this "hyperreligiosity" can appear even in people who deny religious faith. One patient with this trait was an atheist because he felt the clergy were not sufficiently devout; another stated, "God would strike me dead if I were to set foot in church!"; and a third interrupted a church service by going up to the pulpit to debate a theological point. Conventionally religious or not, hyperreligious patients hold profound moral and ethical convictions. In some patients, hyperreligiosity merges with hypergraphia, as in van Gogh, who wrote to Theo from Arles: "I often feel a terrible need of—shall I say the word?—of religion. Then I go out at night to paint the stars."

Two other traits that Geschwind had associated with TLE seemed at first to contradict each other, but they both made sense when Waxman considered each the result of overstimulation by an epileptic scar of the brain region where emotions are controlled. On the one hand, his TLE patients were unusually clingy and dependent, friendly to a fault. They prolonged interactions and conversations beyond the norm, repeatedly telephoning or returning to doctors' offices after appointments, fearful that they had omitted some crucial detail. Gastaut, noting that van Gogh "extended to his few intimates a total, tyrannical love that allowed for no rest, no interruption, no change," called this trait "hypersociability," while Geschwind called it "viscosity," or "stickiness." On the other hand, Waxman and Geschwind observed, their TLE patients felt unusual amounts of anger. Some reported that even an ordinary activity like reading the front page of the morning paper prompted in them such outrage that they were compelled to write letters to the editor several times a week. Their anger occasionally led to violence, sometimes with criminal consequences. One man with TLE had attacked his siblings when he was eighteen. The writer of songs, poems, and aphorisms had assaulted several people and spent years in jail. And the man who dictated his life story to a stenographer reported being easily provoked to rage: he had been discharged from the army for initiating "altercations" and had been arrested for damaging property and assaulting an officer. Although violence can occur during seizures, Waxman and Geschwind found that the vast majority of violent acts perpetrated by people with TLE occurs between, not during, seizures. Moreover, patients' violence is rarely directed toward others; like van Gogh, most people with TLE direct their rage mainly at themselves.

The final trait that Geschwind had mentioned at grand rounds, "altered sexuality," also appeared floridly in van Gogh. Although he boasted to Theo of regular visits to brothels, he admitted that he rarely used prostitutes except as models. He lived for two years with a "stupid" alcoholic beggarwoman and her children not for companionship, he said, but to paint domestic life from experience. Mentioning to Theo in 1888 that he was impotent, he added, "It's all the same to me." He pursued several women who were already married or engaged, including his cousin, whose rejection prompted him to plunge his hand into the flame of a candle, and he failed to pursue the one woman, a neighbor of his parents, who was ever known to fall in love with him. His interest in Gauguin was partly sexual, or "more than a friendship," in the words of Shahram Khoshbin, a neurologist who has studied van Gogh's life. "There can be little doubt," the psychoanalyst Albert J. Lubin added, "that Vincent's wish to live with Gauguin was less a wish for the business partnership of which he wrote than for a passionate love affair." During the time the painters lived together in Arles, Gauguin awakened several times to find van Gogh approaching his bed. "Invariably," Gauguin recalled, "it sufficed for me to say to him very soberly, 'What's the matter, Vincent?' and he would return to his bed without speaking a word and fall into a deep slumber." Gastaut concluded that van Gogh suffered from a "progressive sexual deficiency," or global loss of interest in sex, which worsened during his two-year period of recurring seizures.

Waxman's patients, when queried about their sexuality, reported homosexuality, changes in sexual orientation, transvestism, exhibitionism, pederasty, and fetishism with surprising frequency, all of which suggested a neurological role in sexual preference. One man with TLE was aroused by the sight of a safety pin—a striking result of damage to the emotional part of the brain. Some patients reported cross dressing. Others were strangely promiscuous. For instance, a young man who said he had never experienced lust devised an experiment to discover the nature of sex: he initiated relations with a series of women of widely varying ages. Finding none of them arousing, he took men, animals, and even children to bed. Abandoning the project as a failure, he returned to his comfortable, chaste state.

In most cases of TLE, in fact, patients are "hyposexual," feeling less than ordinary amounts of sexual longing. In one study, more than half of fifty randomly selected TLE patients were hyposexual, reporting sexual feelings less than once a month and sexual activity only once or twice a year. People who develop TLE as adults, Waxman noted, often describe a sudden reduction in sexual interest; while this rarely troubles the patient, it often bothers the spouse. At first Waxman viewed this trait as different from the others, because it usually involves a diminution, rather than an intensification, of an ordinary trait.

Geschwind resolved the apparent inconsistency by theorizing that when sexuality is reduced with TLE, the ordinary function enhanced by the activity of the epileptic scar is the inhibition against sex, which appears to have a physiological basis.

As the evidence mounted to suggest a link between these traits and TLE, Waxman became convinced that a personality "syndrome"—a set of symptoms not necessarily in themselves indicative of disease—does accompany TLE. This syndrome, which he and Geschwind considered unique to TLE, consists of five traits: hypergraphia, hyperreligiosity, stickiness, aggression, and altered sexuality. Their conjunction in TLE patients marks the traits as symptomatic of the disorder. While the syndrome is not present in every patient, it appeared far too frequently for Waxman to deny its association with TLE. Many of his patients displayed two or three of the traits in striking ways. "The syndrome is not subtle, when you see it," he said. "When I looked at these patients and talked to them more carefully than I had before, I found that, if anything, the syndrome is more profound than Norman Geschwind said."

Having convinced himself of the truth of an idea he had initially dismissed, Waxman determined to collaborate with Geschwind in writing about personality and TLE. The problem was how to avoid the appearance of denigrating people with the disorder. "We were well aware that this was a charged area," Waxman explained, "because epileptics have been misrepresented and mistreated for centuries." The long association between epilepsy and madness, criminal behavior, and a host of unpleasant traits had spawned discrimination against epileptics, which continued well into the twentieth century. Even in the 1970s, some states prevented epileptics from obtaining a marriage license, a driver's license, and equal access to a job. "We asked ourselves, 'What's the responsible thing to do, given that very severe, inappropriate prejudice exists and we don't want to make it worse?'" They decided that the subject, however controversial, was too illuminating to ignore. "Personality change in temporal lobe epilepsy," Geschwind observed, "may well be the most important single set of clues we possess to deciphering the neurological systems that underlie the emotional forces that guide behavior," in nonepileptics as well as in people with TLE.

Starting in 1974, articles on what Waxman and Geschwind dubbed "the interictal behavior syndrome of TLE" appeared in medical journals, under both doctors' names. "Even though the idea was Norman's," Waxman said, "he let me put my name first. He was a very giving chief." The doctors described the syndrome with care: the word *syndrome* indicates that the traits alone do not signify a disorder or disease; and since *ictus* is Greek for "seizure," *interictal* means that the traits occur between seizures, as part of a patient's ongoing personality. The doctors hypothesized that the cause of these traits is not seizures but the underlying brain scar, which causes "hyperconnectivity," or too many and too rapid connections in the emotional part of the brain, producing what Geschwind called "an excessive investment of the environment" with emotional significance. As a result, "external stimuli begin to take on great importance," which leads to "increased concern with philosophical, religious, and cosmic matters" and the desire to record experiences "at great length and in highly charged language." The group of traits first became known as the "interictal personality syndrome" or the "Waxman-Geschwind syndrome," but in 1984, after the unexpected death of Norman Geschwind at age fifty-eight, the syndrome was informally renamed in his honor.

Geschwind's accomplishment lay not in discovering "Geschwind's syndrome" but in giving it widespread recognition. Over the years other doctors had noted the similarities of character among their patients with TLE. Gastaut had written about van Gogh's unusual personality, which the neurologist considered typical of people with TLE, in 1956. Several years earlier, Penfield had described finding in TLE patients frequent "behavior abnormalities" and "minor peculiarities," including "defective memory, nervousness, irritability, outbursts of temper, confusion, depression, and neuroses." A young Frenchman was "overconscientious and given to religious and 'mystical' thinking." An "intelligent businessman" from New Jersey who had parts of his right temporal lobe surgically removed had complained of extreme nervousness and tension. Penfield maintained that "some such description is not unusual in these cases." Even earlier, Jackson had noted that TLE patients often had a distinctive personality, being quick to anger and unusually interested in religion. Many doctors had quietly noted the connection between personality and TLE, but Geschwind was the pioneer in publicizing it.

Throughout his career, Geschwind emphasized the achievements, rather than the impairments, of his patients. He believed that neither TLE nor the syndrome has any effect on intellect. While some observers viewed the traits of Geschwind's syndrome as peculiarities or even character defects, Geschwind refused to place any kind of value on them, negative or positive. He considered them simply alterations of traits that appear, to some degree, in everyone: the sense of significance that impels people to write, draw, and believe in God; the need for human contact; aggression; and sexual longing. He felt that only the intensity of these ordinary traits distinguishes people with TLE from other people. He looked to history for examples of successful adaptation to the syndrome, often repeating the playful remark of his colleague, the psychiatrist John Nemiah, that the Puritans who settled in New England in the seventeenth century, with their inveterate journal writing and strict religious and moral codes, may have had the syndrome. In part to pacify those who might accuse him of criticizing epileptics, Geschwind elucidated the benefits of the syndrome in a famous Russian writer who had epilepsy for more than thirty years.

"One must diagnose Dostoevsky as a sufferer from TLE," Geschwind noted during a lecture in Boston in 1961. He based the diagnosis on statements by doctors who had treated the writer, on his voluminous letters, journals, and novels, and on several biographies. According to Geschwind, Fyodor Mikhailovich Dostoevsky's epilepsy began in his childhood, adolescence, or early adulthood; it worsened during the ten difficult years he spent in prison and exile in Siberia, from 1849 to 1859; and it ceased, inexplicably, in 1877, four years before his death. The specific cause of Dostoevsky's epilepsy was unknown, but the fatal three-hour series of grand mal seizures suffered by his two-year-old son, Alyosha, on May 16, 1878, indicated a familial predisposition.

Geschwind considered TLE to have been a motivational and defining force in Dostoevsky's life and work: "When this tragic disease is visited upon a man of genius, he is able to extract from it a depth of understanding." Seizures and a general deepening of emotional response gave Dostoevsky "a shortcut to apprehension of depth of emotion not readily available. . . . Epilepsy is a central source of themes, personalities, and events" in his books. "It enabled him to see some of the most primitive and powerful sources of human behavior. . . . It was abnormal but it still made him feel deeply an aspect of human response that is essential to a literary artist."

Dostoevsky's seizures occurred periodically, every few months or days. Each one started with an ecstatic feeling which he could not fully describe. "You strong people have no idea of the bliss which epileptics experience in the moments preceding their attacks," he wrote. "For several moments, I have a feeling of happiness which I never experienced in my normal state and which one cannot imagine. It is a complete harmony in myself and in the wide world and this feeling is so sweet, so strong, that, I assure you, for a few seconds of this felicity one could give ten years of his life, indeed his entire life." The rest of the seizure was less pleasant. He felt anguish, dread, and guilt, as if he had committed some "monstrous crime." He saw a blinding flash of light and paused as if searching for a word. With the sensation that his voice belonged not to him but to a nonhuman being that had climbed inside his body, he cried out and lost consciousness for a second or two. Sometimes the epileptic discharge generalized across his brain, producing a secondary grand mal attack. Afterward he could not recall events and conversations that had occurred during the seizure, and he often felt depressed, guilty, and irritable for days.

Dostoevsky exploited these abnormal experiences in his fiction, creating numerous characters with epilepsy, some of whose seizures were transcribed directly from the author's journals. In *The Possessed*, for instance, a character named Kirilov has moments of "eternal harmony," similar to Dostoevsky's own, once or twice a week. "It's nothing earthly," Kirilov says in the novel. "You forgive nothing because there is nothing to forgive. . . . It is much higher than love! What is so terrifying about it is that it's so terribly clear and such gladness. If it went on for more than five seconds, the soul could not endure it and must perish. In those five seconds I live through a lifetime, and I'm ready to give my whole life for them, for it's worth it."

"Take care, Kirilov," another character warns. "I've heard that's just how an epileptic fit begins. An epileptic described to me exactly that preliminary sensation before a fit, exactly as you've done. . . . Be careful, Kirilov—it's epilepsy!"

Laughing softly, Kirilov replies, "There won't be time," an allusion to his plan, later fulfilled, to kill himself.

Prince Myshkin, the saintly title character of *The Idiot* whose eyes possess "that strange expression which makes people realize at the first glance that they are dealing with an epileptic," has experiences similar to Kirilov's. "Suddenly in the midst of sadness, spiritual darkness and oppression, there seemed at moments a flash of light in [Myshkin's] brain, and with extraordinary impetus all his vital forces suddenly began working at their highest tension. The . . . consciousness of self was multiplied ten times. . . . His mind and his heart were flooded with extraordinary light . . . all his anxieties were relieved at once; they were all merged in a lofty calm, full of serene, harmonious joy and hope. . . . These moments were only an extraordinary quickening of self-consciousness . . . and at the same time of the direct sensation of existence in the most intense degree. Since at that second, that is at the very last conscious moment before the fit, he had time to say to himself clearly and consciously: 'Yes, for this moment one might give one's whole life!'"

In Geschwind's view, Dostoevksy's novels portray not only actual seizure states but also the personality syndrome. Many of the author's characters are obsessed with philosophy, mysticism, and morality. Readers of Dostoevsky, according to Geschwind, are "constantly made aware that all events are of great importance and that there are no minor incidents." There is little mention in the novels of sex. Most striking is the violence of the plots. For instance, the hero of *The Gambler* insults people without provocation. Without apparent premeditation, the narrator of *Notes from Underground* creates an unpleasant scene at a reunion. The central character in *Crime and Punishment* kills an old woman pawnbroker with a hatchet, and *The Brothers Karamazov* revolves around the murder of a father by a son who happens to be epileptic. In *The Possessed*, a man impulsively pinches the nose of an official and later bites a governor's ear. "There can be little doubt," Geschwind said, "of the novels' mirroring in considerably enlarged extent Dostoevsky's own behavior in life." Dostoevsky did have attacks of rage, according to family and friends, which clustered in the days following seizures and contrasted with his normally sweet disposition. The author's "cosmic concerns," prolixity, "constant intensity of emotion," humorlessness, and apparent asexuality until his middle thirties further suggested to the neurologist that Dostoevsky himself had Geschwind's syndrome.

It was Geschwind's belief that the creative work of people with the syndrome is no less worthy of admiration because of its association with a neurological disorder. Apparently Dostoevsky agreed. Prince Myshkin, his fictional alter ego, worries that the moment of religious ecstasy he feels in seizures is suspect because of its source in epilepsy. "Thinking of that moment later, when he was all right again, [Myshkin] often said to himself that all these gleams and flashes of the highest sensation of life and self-consciousness, and therefore also of the highest form of existence, were nothing but disease, the interruption of the normal condition; and if so, it was not at all the highest form of being, but on the contrary must be reckoned the lowest."

After much consideration, Myshkin nevertheless decides that his ecstatic moments are real and true, that his "highest sensation of life" cannot be dismissed or explained away because it arises from a disorder. "What if it is disease?" muses Dostoevsky's prince. "What does it matter that it is an abnormal intensity, if the result, if the minute of sensation, remembered and analysed afterwards in health, turns out to be the acme of harmony and beauty, and gives a feeling, unknown and undivined till then, of completeness, of proportion . . . and of ecstatic devotional merging in the highest synthesis of life?!"

In the larger population of patients, Geschwind's syndrome has a wide range of effects, proving a boon in some people, and a curse in others. Hyperreligiosity can be seen as piety in one person, obsessiveness in another. Stickiness can appear as overdependence or loyalty. Hypergraphia can result in worthless scribblings or such masterpieces as Dostoevsky's novels and van Gogh's late landscapes. The end to which a person directs her intensified emotions is subject to unknown laws. In general, Geschwind speculated, the syndrome intensifies whatever emotional tendency is already present. A sensitive person becomes volatile. A controlled person rigidifies. A spiritual person writes a religious tome. The change is not intrinsically good or bad:

someone with Geschwind's syndrome may be a criminal or a model citizen. Donald Schomer, a neurologist who worked with Geschwind in the early 1980s, concluded that TLE generally affects personality by pushing people to emotional extremes: a patient's emotions can be muted or enhanced. "More often than not," Schomer said, "patients with TLE tend to react in the emotional world either excessively or in a blunted fashion." In a sense, people with TLE are like everyone else—only more so.

CHAPTER THREE

Ordinary People

On Sunday, December 15, 1974, in the early afternoon, Charlie Higgins set out across his lawn. A slight, wiry man of fifty-three with a full head of straw-gray hair, Charlie wore a country lawyer's weekend suit: L. L. Bean hunting boots, faded chinos, a flannel shirt, and a worn, wine-colored down vest. He headed toward the woods behind his house, where a storm had downed several maple trees, slow-burning hardwoods that would, he knew, make fine fireplace logs. In his right hand was a four-foot cross-cut saw.

At this moment, Charlie had achieved pretty much everything for which he ever hoped. Born in Indianapolis in 1921, the fourth and last child of an insurance man and an amateur singer, Charlie had come east to attend Princeton and then Harvard Law School. While serving in the Navy during the Second World War, he had met and married a Boston Yankee, with whom he had settled in this pleasant Vermont town in the late 1940s. Locals came to know Charlie, a winker with a fondness for the phrase "You bet," as a "true Vermonter—industrious, says what he means, caring, and does a lot of good works quietly." The "dean" of local lawyers, he was a founding partner in a prominent firm and someone on whom neighbors called to settle disputes. His civic service included several years each as a Rotary Club president, state senator, and county judge. He ran several miles daily, and he was in excellent health.

That Sunday in December, he and his wife, Fran, had eaten breakfast early and gone to church, where he sang in the choir and served on the board. Afterward, at home, they had done the chores with their children, Rachel, who was home on vacation from college, and Michael, a high-school junior. At noon the family had convened for lunch. Fran had cleared the table, Rachel and Michael had gone out with friends, and Charlie— who dislikes the racket made by power saws—had sharpened his antique crosscut saw.

Now, as he neared the line where his yard, which was covered in new snow, meets the woods, he turned to wave at Fran, who was visible in the kitchen window. Then he smiled and disappeared into the woods.

It is easy to imagine getting lost here, but Charlie knew every turn and fallen branch along the way. He had cut the trails himself. To the east, he could see the purple-gray ridge of mountains that he and his family often climbed. Between the mountains and the woods, a valley descends. On one side of the valley, through the bare trees, he could make out a row of houses, one of the developments springing up in rural New England. The northernmost white house belonged to his family doctor.

Deeper into the woods, the land rises slightly. The firs are denser and the maples younger. The storm had strewn slender white birches across the path. At a scattering of branches, Charlie stopped. Beneath him lay the trunk of a sugar maple, twenty-five feet long. Standing a log's length from one end of it, he bowed his head and began to saw. The work felt good. Charlie concentrated on the back-and-forth motion of the saw. With the exertion, his breathing became heavy and fast.

Suddenly, without warning, he felt "funny." It seemed that his consciousness had intensified and doubled, as though he were dreaming while awake. He felt he was in two worlds at once: the logical, real world of ordinary experience; and the irrational, larger-than-life world of dreams. The experience might have seemed imaginary, except for the unpleasant physical sensation accompanying it—"a bodily sense of malaise" consisting of queasiness, nausea, and an odd pressure behind his temples.

Charlie knew nothing of the nature of this state of mind, but he did know that he had experienced it before. It had occurred every year or so during the previous ten years: once at a Rotary lunch, once while driving himself home, and several times while exerting himself physically—skiing, shoveling, or chopping wood. Until the past year, when these momentary experiences began to occur more frequently, he had kept them to himself. Then the previous winter, while shoveling snow with his son, Charlie had complained of "a funny feeling." Another day, while downhill skiing with Fran, he had told her, "I feel a little out of it. It's that feeling of being in another world that I sometimes have." In the summer, sitting on his back steps with his brother-in-law after a driving game of tennis, Charlie had murmured, "I feel dizzy," and held his head. There was never a visible sign of anything wrong. Fran, who had always considered her husband "a daydreamer, a little absentminded," didn't worry about these occasional feelings. And when Charlie had described them to his family doctor at an annual physical examination, the doctor brushed them aside. They didn't sound serious. Still, no one knew what they were.

In the woods, Charlie continued sawing as long as he could, until his growing nausea forced him to stop. He lowered his head, waiting for the feeling to go away. As his breathing and heart rate slowed, the strange sensations subsided. Thinking that the brisk air had cleared his mind, Charlie took a deep breath and resumed his task.

Moments later the feeling returned, coming over him now like a wave. In addition to the woods around him, the tree trunk at his feet, and the crosscut saw in his hands, he was conscious of another world. He felt he was waking slowly from a vivid dream; the waking was greatly delayed, leaving him suspended between reality and the dream.

In a kind of daze, he began to walk. He had no idea where he was or where he was going, but he did know that he could not find his way home. His own woods were unfamiliar.

Nearly an hour later, back at the house, Fran was dozing in an armchair by the fireplace, a novel open on her lap and a cold cup of tea at her side. At three o'clock the chimes of the grandfather clock woke her, and she cried, "Charlie!" There was no response. She went to the kitchen window to see if he was in the yard, but no one was there. She was surprised he was taking so long. He had suggested that they go cross-country skiing that afternoon, so he should have been back by now; night falls early in midwinter in Vermont. Fran put on her wool vest and suede jacket and marched out into the woods.

Minutes later, she heard a faint voice. She called out, but there was no reply. The voice kept on chattering, as if engaged in a conversation with itself. Fran hastened in its direction. The moment she saw Charlie, she knew something was wrong. Her articulate, focused husband stood off the path, in the snow, mumbling to himself, his crosscut saw in his hand. He looked disconnected and unaware. She approached him and asked, "What's wrong?"

"Something's wrong," he acknowledged vaguely. "I don't know where I am. I can't find my way back home."

"Is this something you've experienced before?"

Charlie nodded. Oh my gosh, Fran thought, this is one of his episodes of being in his dream world. She took the saw from him and led him home. He followed docilely, asking her after every few steps where he was. Over and over she told him, and each time he forgot. Despite this confusion, he didn't seem upset; his emotion and his intellect seemed to have split apart. He was like a robot, his emotions and memory temporarily turned off.

At the house, warm and scented with the pot roast that she had left in the oven, Fran brought him to the sofa and sat him down. "Do you know where you are now?" she asked. He said no. She repeatedly asked him this question. After about ten minutes, he finally told her he was home.

Still, he wasn't himself. He couldn't recall what he had been doing in the woods. She explained that he had been cutting firewood with his crosscut saw, and he replied, "I was using a crosscut saw. Why was I using a crosscut saw?" A piece of his memory was gone.

Time passed, and Fran's worry grew. Charlie's episodes had never lasted more than several minutes, but this one was already at least half an hour long. She dialed the doctor's number. A recording announced that he was out of town and that another doctor would handle his emergency calls. Fran decided to wait a little longer.

At four o'clock, the Charlie she knew still hadn't returned.

She called the local hospital, asked for the doctor on call, and described to him what had happened. He instructed her to drive Charlie to the hospital. She helped her husband into the passenger seat, buckled his seat belt, and started the car. At first, Charlie was aware that his wife was driving him somewhere. A minute later, his memory stopped. He remained fully conscious, but his mind, which for two hours had been poised between the real world and the dream, now slipped over into the dream world, where memories can be neither stored nor retrieved. Whatever had turned on his memory abnormally in the woods had now shut it off entirely. From now on, he would be amnesic until the episode ended.

At the hospital, the doctor admitted him to a private room. Charlie undressed and got into bed. He remained calm, "but he sounded like a broken record," according to Fran. "He kept babbling, 'I was using a crosscut saw. Why was I using a crosscut saw?'" The doctor asked Charlie the standard neurological questions that determine a patient's mental state: What is your name? Where are you? What day is today? What year is it? Who is the President of the United States? "He knew who he was but not where he was or why he was there," according to Rachel, who had returned home to find a scribbled note from her mother and then rushed to the hospital. Nineteen-year-old Rachel, who is now an electroencephalographer, was already interested in medicine and the brain. "At the hospital, Dad had a memory span of about thirty seconds," she observed. "He would ask us a question, and thirty seconds later he'd ask the same question." His memory of the more distant past was also impaired. He couldn't remember the name of his daughter's college. Although Gerald Ford was President, Eisenhower was the last President that Charlie could recall. Rachel observed in her father the same splitting of intellect and emotion that Fran had seen in the woods. "Dad *knew* something was wrong with him, but he couldn't *sense* it."

News of Charlie's trouble spread through the town. The doctor's wife contacted the Higginses' minister, who came to Charlie's room and was deeply troubled by what he found. "Charlie is a very precise, careful, think-before-he-speaks kind of person," the minister said later, "and yet here he was acting in a manner totally out of character. He could respond quite coherently to our talk about his activities in the woods—cutting trees and wandering around—but the minute you stopped talking about it he had absolutely no memory of what anyone had just said. He couldn't even remember that he couldn't remember!"

Charlie's symptoms especially worried Fran. She feared that they were caused by a tumor or a stroke, which could damage tissue, perhaps permanently, in the brain region controlling memory and consciousness.

To everyone's surprise, after a few hours and without any treatment, Charlie began to improve. His memory of the remote past gradually filled in. After dinner, he could remember everything except the last several hours. He stopped repeating whatever was said to him, he went to sleep, and Fran agreed to go home for the night. Early the next morning, she was awakened by the telephone. The minister was calling from the hospital. "Charlie's fine," he said. "He's with it again." When Fran arrived, she discovered that her husband was "his old self." Charlie confessed that he still felt "confused and a little dull," so he spent another night at the hospital. Tuesday morning, feeling fine, he went to work. Other than the "big blank" in his memory, which lasted from the time he "blacked out" on the way to the hospital until the moment, six or eight hours later, when he "came to" in his hospital bed, there were no aftereffects. As Fran said, "He appeared perfectly normal right away."

Charlie's rapid recovery, his limited amnesia, and his description of a dreamy state with head and gastrointestinal pain indicated to the doctor that he had had a TLE seizure, probably caused by hyperventilation while sawing. Hyperventilation reduces the oxygen to the brain, destabilizing electrical activity and increasing the chance of seizing in anyone, especially in someone prone to epilepsy. The doctor suspected that epileptic activity in the brain region controlling Charlie's memory had caused the mix of memories that composes a dreamy state. That mental state and the accompanying "bodily sense of malaise," which is another characteristic manifestation of TLE, had abated when Charlie first stopped sawing, due to increased oxygen to his brain, but the seizure had come back in full force when he returned to his labor. Eventually, the doctor thought, epileptic brain activity had shut off Charlie's memory, causing the hours of seizural amnesia. Thinking that the word *epilepsy* would alarm Charlie and his family, however, the doctor did not share his suspicions with them. Instead, he suggested that Charlie consult a neurologist and have an EEG.

At home, it was easy for the Higginses to forget that anything was wrong. Charlie is known for his equanimity, and the family followed his lead. They celebrated Christmas and New Year's as usual. Not until January 3, more than two weeks after the episode in the woods, did Charlie and Fran drive to Rutland, Vermont, to see the nearest neurologist.

Margaret Waddington made the same diagnosis as the other doctor, but her manner was far more straightforward. The neurologist was known for her candor; she also sensed Charlie's intelligence and ability to handle bad news. "He is," she wrote in her notes, "a most delightful person, very friendly, alert, well oriented, and in no distress." Immediately after hearing his description of brief, intermittent attacks of confusion, dizziness, vague pain, and amnesia over several years, she told him, "These episodes of altered states of consciousness surely sound like a seizure disorder, probably temporal lobe." To confirm her diagnosis, she said, she would give him an EEG, which detects epileptic activity in the brain. She led him into a room containing an EEG machine, instructed him to lie on a stretcher, and glued several electrodes to his scalp over his temporal lobes. Aware that seizing during the test increases the chance of finding abnormal activity on an EEG, she told him to hyperventilate, imitating the strenuous exercise that had prompted past episodes. Charlie hyperventilated, but he didn't seize. Waddington turned on the machine and interpreted the record of his brain activity as it appeared on the page. "That's terrible!" she exclaimed upon finding strikingly abnormal activity even in the absence of seizures. "Oh, my goodness, look at *that!*" she added. Charlie was relieved that Fran was not in the room. "I don't alarm easily," he said later, "but if Fran had heard Waddington reacting to the irregularities in my EEG, she would have had a fit."

"Oh, that's terrible," Waddington continued. "I think you have a lesion, and it might well be malignant!"

This was Waddington's greatest fear—not the TLE itself, but the likelihood that a tumor was its cause. Epilepsy that develops slowly and relatively late in life is often caused by the pressure of a slow-growing tumor, as it was in Ruth Penfield's case. When Waddington had examined Charlie, she had asked numerous questions about his early life and medical history; based on his answers, she had ruled out most of the likely causes of epilepsy—head injury, encephalitis, meningitis, epilepsy in the family, birth trauma, childhood seizures, and drug abuse—none of which Charlie or Fran thought applied to him. The only remaining explanation for his TLE seemed to be a brain tumor. This dire possibility was supported by a "disconcerting" physical finding Waddington had made during her test of his neurological functions. When she had tapped tendons in his arms and legs, his reflexes were unequal, those on the left being abnormally brisk. This left-sided reflex problem suggested an abnormality, such as a tumor, in the right side of the brain, which controls the body's left side. As a "tentative diagnosis," the neurologist wrote in Charlie's chart, "Tumor suspect, until proven otherwise." Actually, she confided to Charlie, she didn't suspect he had a tumor; she was convinced of it.

This ominous news terrified Fran when she heard it on the way home. "That was when the fear really began," she recalls. "Of course, my nature is to worry." Charlie, characteristically, wasn't upset. Faced with the prospect of imminent death, he was "philosophical," according to his wife. Charlie agrees, "I didn't lose sleep over it. I wasn't afraid. I don't know why. Maybe it was my religious faith. My general philosophical view is that I've lived a very good and happy life, and if I were taken, I'd have no complaints."

To treat Charlie's seizures, Waddington prescribed anticonvulsant medications, which reduced the seizures' intensity and frequency. In the hope of locating the suspected tumor, she recommended a complete neurological workup, including skull X rays and sophisticated brain scans that were not available nearby. Charlie drove to the Dartmouth Medical School for a CAT scan, a computerized device that pictures internal body tissues. A CAT scan of his brain, however, showed no evidence of a tumor. As his doctors still sought a tumor, Charlie spent five days in Burlington, at the University of Vermont Medical Center, having further brain tests, some of which are invasive and painful. All the tests were negative; no tumor was unearthed.

Without any visible sign of a tumor, Waddington was stumped as to why Charlie had developed an epileptic scar. But the lack of an explanation is not unusual, she reassured him; doctors are frequently unable in cases of TLE to determine the specific cause of the scar, which can be as forgettable an event in a patient's life as a childhood fall on the head. If Charlie wanted to learn more about what was wrong in his brain, she added, he could undergo a neurosurgical evaluation at a major medical center. At this point, Charlie balked. His seizures did not seem serious enough to justify allowing a surgeon to cut into his brain. The risks of surgery, he thought, far outweighed the potential benefits.

Several months later, Thomas Donaghy, a neurosurgeon and family friend whom the Higginses consulted, came up with a theory about the cause of Charlie's disorder. In a roundabout way, according to Donaghy, Charlie got TLE because of a raccoon.

In the summer of 1932, when he was twelve, Charlie had spent two weeks at a Boy Scout camp—the first time he had slept even a night away from home. Upon his return, he ran straight for the backyard, where he kept a couple of pet raccoons in a chicken-wire cage. The pair were accustomed to being fed peanuts from Charlie's hand every afternoon, and for two weeks no one had brought any peanuts. Now, in his excitement, Charlie had forgotten to stuff peanuts in his pocket.

As usual, he unlocked the door of the cage and climbed right in with the raccoons. The male dove for the pocket where the peanuts usually were. Finding no food, the animal went wild and attacked the boy, biting his hands and elbows and tearing his clothes. Eyes bulging in anger, the raccoon ripped the cage door off its hinges and jammed it against the frame, locking Charlie in. Hearing his screams, his father sprinted from the house to find Charlie bloody and in shock. The father shouted the animals to the rear of the cage, forced the door open, and lifted out his son. He lay the boy on the backseat of his car and drove to a farmhouse where a doctor lived. They cleaned Charlie's wounds. Fearing that the raccoon was rabid, the doctor administered the Pasteur treatment, which consisted of injecting a small amount of rabies into Charlie's blood, through his abdomen. The procedure guaranteed a light case of rabies fever, as against the fatal risk of full-fledged rabies.

Predictably, the boy's temperature rose dramatically. A terrible fever kept him in bed for a month. At times he was delirious, hallucinating that his bed was floating around the room. At the end of the month, he began to regain his strength, and soon he resumed his normal activities. He seemed fine. For decades to come, there was no reason to suspect that the incident had left any trace but the slender scar, the outline of a raccoon's jaw, on one of Charlie's palms.

Donaghy suspected that there was a second, invisible scar. According to the neurosurgeon, the rabies vaccination had given Charlie encephalitis, a viral infection to the brain. This infection had probably affected his hippocampus, a structure deep inside the temporal lobes to which the rabies virus frequently goes. Like TLE, rabies is associated with personality change: people with rabies become anxious, fearful, and aggressive; and the word *rabies* comes from the Latin for "madness" or "rage." The infection had caused the fever, which in turn had left a scar on Charlie's brain. Some years later, that lesion had become the site of abnormal electrical activity, which had developed into little seizures in Charlie's forties and culminated in the big seizure in the woods.

Lacking evidence suggestive of another likely cause, Charlie's doctors accepted Donaghy's explanation for his TLE. Keith Edwards, the neurologist who took over Charlie's care when Waddington retired, observed, "I don't think he had true rabies, which is uniformly fatal. But the rabies vaccine, which gave lots of people a little encephalitis back then, probably did induce encephalitis, which has been known to cause epilepsy. Charlie's distinctly unusual EEG—a rapid frontal beta pattern that we sometimes see in encephalitis—is actually objective evidence that his TLE is probably related to the vaccine."

Even without the history of the vaccine, Edwards found it reasonable to assume that Charlie had a minor case of encephalitis as a child. "Many children," the neurologist noted, "have a flu virus, get a little encephalitis, run a 105-degree fever and are up all night, delirious, and maybe have a seizure—the kid stiffens and shakes for a few minutes, and the mother doesn't know it's a seizure—and they're fine in a week or two. That happens to about half of all kids. So if Charlie hadn't had the vaccine I'd assume he'd had an infection like that, which was missed, and that it caused a little scar on his brain."

More than fifteen years after his diagnosis, Charlie is among the lucky minority of people with TLE, because the effect of seizures on his life is slight. Past seventy, he is in far better shape than most American men his age—his body muscular and thin, his crinkled face still boyishly open. Charlie continues, despite his TLE, to function at a high level. He works full time at his law firm, handling wills and real estate, which he prefers to litigation and courtroom work. Now that their children are grown, he and Fran live by themselves; in their spare time they travel, play bridge, and tend their fruit trees, raspberries, and herbs. Since 1982 he has been on an anticonvulsant drug called Tegretol, which controls his TLE well.

"I can't remember when I last had a seizure," he said one recent autumn, standing in his yard, a rake in his hand. Before his doctors prescribed Tegretol, he had had a few seizures as disruptive as the one in the woods, except that he now knew what they were. In the summer of 1976, while working in the garden, he momentarily lost consciousness and found himself on the ground; four years later, while cutting down a lilac bush, he had a dreamy state in which he wandered about the yard, uncertain where he was and what he was doing. But since he started taking Tegretol, all his seizures have been "passing things," brief dreamy states, hallucinations of flashing lights, or an unpleasant light-headedness that, typical of TLE, is difficult for him to put into words. These seizures, which occur only once or twice a year, "don't interrupt the normal flow of activity." He has learned to stop whatever he is doing when he senses a seizure coming. If he lies down for fifteen minutes, the feeling usually goes away. At work, his longtime secretary teases him for lying on his office floor from time to time. "He'll often say he's having a funny feeling of something coming on," the secretary says, "but I can't see it, and it doesn't last long. It's hard to believe he really has epilepsy, because he's the same as he ever was, busy all the time."

Indeed the changes in his life since his diagnosis have been few. Three times a day he must take an anticonvulsant pill—a modest dose, according to Edwards, whom he sees briefly once a year. The results of Charlie's last EEG, in 1981, though strikingly abnormal, were just the same as the one Edwards did the year before, suggesting that his seizure focus was not spreading. If he stopped taking the drug, he could have "episodes of confusion, amnesia, and semi-automatic activity" every week or month, Edwards said. Because alcohol and lack of sleep have caused Charlie to seize on occasion, he no longer drinks, and he makes sure that he gets enough sleep. His crosscut saw has hung, rusting, on a nail in his well-ordered shed since his seizure in the woods. "I gave up forest work after that," he said. "Oh, I'll split a log or two for kindling now and then, but I never put in anything like the effort I was making that day in 1974." Since the diagnosis of his TLE, he burns coal, rather than wood, in the stove that heats his house.

TLE also prompted Charlie to give up downhill skiing. In March 1975, a few months after his diagnosis and just weeks after he started taking Dilantin, one of the first anticonvulsants that Waddington prescribed, he was making fast runs down a local mountain by himself. In the afternoon, as he ascended the mountain on the chairlift, a dreamy state began. Chances are, he says, he had hyperventilated: "I held my breath a lot when I skied." The dreamy state consisted of a flashback that he cannot recall, the familiar "funny feeling" in his head and stomach, and the aura of unreality. He managed to get off the chairlift and start skiing down the mountain, but the seizural sensations intensified. When he reached the bottom, he had no idea where he was. He questioned strangers, news of his distress spread among the skiers, and a local doctor led him to the lodge. One of his law partners, who happened to be on the slopes that day, drove him home. Charlie's teenage son, who was in the driveway practicing jumpshots, at first thought that his straight-laced father was inexplicably stoned. "Then Dad told me he was having a bout," Michael said, "that he might repeat himself, and to please bear with him. Other than his being so dazed, though, it seemed as though nothing was wrong. He's always been so able to convey a sense of calm about his TLE that I've never really worried about it."

When Charlie described this extended dreamy state to Waddington, she switched him to a different anticonvulsant, phenobarbital. Because of the risk of hyperventilation triggering more seizures, she also ordered him not to ski downhill. A dutiful patient, Charlie hasn't skied down a mountain since that day.

Going to another extreme that his physician never recommended, Charlie has for several years generally avoided sexual activity. A year after his diagnosis, he mentioned to Waddington that he had experienced a "loss of libido," which he thought might be a side effect of the anticonvulsant he was taking at the time. Waddington reassured him that to her knowledge phenobarbital did not reduce sexual interest; she did not mention to him that TLE itself is associated with altered interest in sex. During the next few years, he had several seizures immediately following intercourse, triggered, he assumed, by the heavy breathing that is natural to the act. For fear of hyperventilating, he said, he is now "less interested" than before in sex.

Still, he participates in sports that cause heavy breathing, including tennis, which induced a seizure in the past. He plays basketball in warm weather; he skis cross-country in winter; and he runs every day of the year. Although his wife worries that while running he may seize and forget the way home, this has never happened. "The reason," he guessed, "is that my breathing is constant and measured when I run." His doctor is confident that Fran's concern is unwarranted, saying that Charlie is unlikely to seize during this kind of exercise as long as he takes the anticonvulsant. Charlie bristles at his wife's anxious attempts to restrict his activities, but he acknowledges that his disorder is harder on her than on him. In deference to her, when running he always wears a belt pouch containing his name and address, which she gave him one Christmas after his diagnosis.

The only other difference Charlie has noticed since his diagnosis is a slight personality change. He had always been focused and careful, a little compulsive, and in the early 1980s, at his annual neurological examination, he reported that this trait had intensified during the previous few years, making him "excessively verbal and detailed." While researching cases at work, for instance, he found himself obsessed with minor points. In conversation, his wife observed, he went on even longer than before, so that polite listeners couldn't always stifle their yawns. Charlie wondered if this change was related to his epilepsy. Edwards thought it wasn't. Charlie, who had read medical articles about TLE and personality change, was relieved. "I understand that some people with TLE get violent and aggressive and fanatically religious," he said. "I sure wouldn't look forward to that."

Other than this vague, unrealized fear of dramatic personality change, Charlie has had little to worry about as a result of his TLE. "I've never felt my epilepsy was a big deal at all," he said. "I never felt the weight of being handicapped or disabled. I can function without any problems; for all intents and purposes, I'm perfectly normal. For a long time I didn't even realize that 'epilepsy' could be a terrible label. I was a demonstration that nothing was wrong. People think that TLE is frightening, but mine is minor enough that it's not really disturbing. The doctors aren't sure of the long-term effects of Tegretol, but it hasn't had any effect on me yet. And my health insurance covers most of the cost." Charlie considers himself fortunate compared to people with other forms of epilepsy. Several years ago at a cocktail party he witnessed a grand mal seizure for the first time. Across the room a woman sipped from her drink and then fell backward to the floor. Not knowing what was wrong, Charlie ran over to help. When the rescue squad arrived, an emergency medical technician asked the woman if she took any medications. "Dilantin," she replied. Charlie thought, "Oh, that's what that was—a classic convulsive attack. By gosh, if she can live with that, I can't worry about my situation."

In Charlie's case, TLE has been delicately superimposed on a placid, satisfying life. His most difficult experiences came early, during the disorienting seizures prior to diagnosis and the brief period when a life-threatening tumor seemed likely to be their cause, but even these did not cause any sleepless nights. In this respect, Charlie is unusual. For most people with TLE, the trauma of the diagnosis is only the beginning of a lengthy trial. As Jill, an executive in her thirties, said a few years after her seizures began, "TLE banged into my life, and it hasn't let up since."

In an office high in a Boston skyscraper, Jill Rasmussen leaned over her spotless desk, furiously proofreading a report. After several years in the personnel departments of headhunting and consulting firms, she was now the director of personnel for a large corporation, in charge of the professional lives of a thousand employees and a multimillion-dollar budget. On this day, Jill, a slight woman with short blonde hair, blue eyes, and manicured nails, wore a black-and-white wool suit, silk blouse, and pearls.

"Damn," she muttered, finding an error in the report. "I knew I shouldn't have done this in a hurry." She ground out her cigarette and tapped another from the pack. For perhaps the millionth time she thought, "This job is like being pecked to death by ducks."

As if to bear out this sentiment, someone rapped on her door. Jill called, "Come in," and a man about her age, an assistant to a vice president with whom she had recently disagreed, poked his head into her office. He began to plead on behalf of his boss. Calmly, Jill said of the boss, "He can't talk me out of it, because I don't think I'm wrong." She paused. "Now I'll give him one more chance before I do something he probably won't like."

Her phone rang. A corporate auditor wanted a list of all employees' names, titles, and job descriptions. He wanted it now. She would get to it when she could, she told him sweetly. She had interviews with several job candidates scheduled for the afternoon.

A woman knocked, entered, and issued a long-winded complaint about a colleague. Jill listened for the problem's gist, consoled the woman, and went back to her report.

A middle-aged man stopped in the doorway. Looking up, Jill gave him a radiant smile. "You know what I need from you?" she said. "It's been almost a year and a half—" The man apologized and went to get the information she wanted.

Her phone rang again. Her secretary had a question about her schedule. As they talked, the company's president leaned into Jill's office, saw that she was on the phone, and left. Minutes later, Jill's secretary buzzed to say that the president was on the line. Jill picked up the phone and said, "How's it going?" The president was looking for the records of a former employee. Hearing the employee's name, Jill said, "Golly, I remember *him*. When do you need it—end of the day?" The president said he did. "End of the *day*?" Jill repeated, feigning disbelief. "OK, I'll have my secretary do it." She added, "When you get a chance, I want to talk to you about the memo you sent on salaries."

On another typical day, at four o'clock, Jill was alone in her office. The day's interviews done, she sat reviewing her notes. Suddenly, she couldn't concentrate. The words she was reading held no meaning for her. She went back over the last few lines in vain. Something far more powerful than her notes was on her mind, "an awful feeling of absolute panic and fear." For no apparent reason, she felt certain that "something really bad" was about to happen. This global, nonspecific terror immobilized her, demanding all the energy and concentration she had. It seemed to come from somewhere deep inside her where she could not reason with herself. Even though the terror was without external basis, she experienced it as though it were utterly justified and true.

This panic, she knew, was a seizure, something like the dread van Gogh occasionally felt. Her doctors had explained to her that epileptic discharge in the part of her brain that controls fear can cause a panic attack. Unfortunately, her knowledge that the feeling is really a seizure does not lessen the intensity of the experience. Each time it happens, it feels horrifically real; the seizure presents itself as actual, impending doom. If one of these panic attacks were to last longer than a few hours, she believes, she would have no choice but to kill herself.

In this case, she prepared to wait out the seizure. She buzzed her secretary and instructed her, in as normal a voice as she could muster, to handle all calls. She rose, steadied herself, and closed her office door. Falling back into her chair, she lit a cigarette; during seizures, nicotine has a calming effect on her.

An hour later, the building began to empty. "See you tomorrow," people called as they departed. No one noticed Jill, frozen in her office.

At about six o'clock, in a nearby office, the corporation counsel, Ted Brownson, wrapped up his work and decided to look in on Jill before going home. A married, suburban homeowner, Ted finds her "much less conventional" than him, but also entertaining, smart, and remarkably adept at her job. "She can interview fifteen people in five hours," he raves. While Ted and Jill don't socialize after hours, they talk a lot at work. He feels protective of her, considering himself rare among her friends in that he has both feet on the ground. "Jill doesn't have many people she can depend on," he says, "but I'm one."

Knocking on her door, he was surprised to get no response. She usually works even later than he does. He knocked again, waited, then opened the door. The office was thick with cigarette smoke. Behind the shiny desk, Jill sat staring into a void. Her face looked troubled, and her eyes did not move.

"What's wrong?" Ted asked.

"I'm afraid," she murmured. She could say nothing more. During a panic attack, even speaking makes her afraid.

"What are you afraid of?"

"I'm afraid."

Ted's first thought was that he had frightened her. But this didn't make sense: she had trusted him for years. Then he remembered that she had mentioned having panic attacks, a result of some kind of seizure disorder. Ted, who had never heard of TLE, was skeptical of the whole business. He didn't think that all the problems she described—not only panic attacks but also bouts of anxiety, confusion, stomach pain, dizziness, and forgetfulness—could be caused by epilepsy. For him, as for many people, epilepsy consists only of grand mal seizures: "It's cut and dried. Epileptics bounce up and down, and you have to put a cork in their mouth." (This recommendation, once intended to prevent people from swallowing their tongues during seizures, is no longer advised, since tongue swallowing is rare in any kind of seizure.) As Ted knows, Jill has never had a grand mal seizure. Most of the time she seems "quite normal." However, at about a third of the meetings that they attend together, "when we get to the issue of personnel and why certain things aren't being done, Jill tunes out." Her sentences become jumbled, she looks lost and bleary eyed, and most unusual, she doesn't smile. To Ted, this seems like a performance. "I wonder if it's because of the substance of the meeting or because of her seizures. How much of what she's experiencing is strictly emotional? I mean, I could have a head cold and convince myself I'm on my death bed." As is typical of people unfamiliar with TLE, he suspects that her seizures are a screen for a psychological problem she can't address. What the problem is, he doesn't know.

Now, faced with this strange behavior in her office, he asked how he could help. "I don't know," she whispered. "I'm afraid." He offered to drive her home. She shook her head and said, "I'm afraid to leave." He encouraged her to talk about what was bothering her, to no avail. Finally, not knowing what else to do, he decided to go home. She was relieved. Her seizural fear cannot be talked out. No one can help her during a panic attack, so she prefers to be left alone.

At eight o'clock, she found she had the energy to make a phone call. The seizure must have waned, for an hour earlier she had been too afraid even to pick up the phone. She dialed the number of Beth Israel Hospital, where her neuropsychologist, Paul Spiers, often worked late. Her voice strained, Jill told Spiers that she was having a panic attack. He suggested an extra dose of the anticonvulsant that she had been taking for a few years. She hung up, dug a vial of Dilantin from her purse, and swallowed a pill.

An hour later, her panic had abated: the seizure had ended. Exhausted from the ordeal, Jill called a cab to drive her home. At the row house where she lives alone, she unlocked the door, climbed the stairs, and dropped onto her bed. When she awoke the next morning, her shoes and coat were still on.

TLE has hit Jill harder than it hit Charlie. While his seizures began in middle age, when he was established in his career and surrounded by a supportive family, hers developed while she was young, uncertain of her professional future, and alone. In her early thirties, with the arc of her life only partly drawn, she was confronted with the anxieties, loneliness, and fear brought on by a chronic illness. Also unlike Charlie, whose seizures quickly responded well to drugs, Jill is among the many people with TLE—25 percent, according to doctors, and 65 percent, according to the patients themselves—for whom drugs do not adequately control seizures. Her doctors tried several anticonvulsants during the years following her diagnosis, but she continued to seize. It seemed that she was always trying a new drug or, as she developed a tolerance to it, watching an old drug lose its effect. Even with the more effective drugs, her symptoms waxed and waned. In general, the bad periods outnumbered the good periods, and even the latter were not as good as the life she had known before. "They're acceptable," she said, "but they're not how I want to spend the rest of my life." In a bad week she averaged three or four seizures a day. Among her various seizure states, the worst were the panic attacks, which occurred about four or five times a year. Like the rest of her seizures, panic attacks came at irregular intervals, without warning. "Seizures have minds of their own," she said. "I can be cruising along, minding my own business, and then this awful feeling just comes over me in a flash." The unpredictability of seizures prompted her to call TLE "a sneaky disease. It creeps around you, and then it's *got* you for a while."

TLE first "got" Jill in July 1983, the summer of her thirty-first year. While shopping in a furniture store with her friend Norma, who was then her apartment mate, Jill realized that she was lost. She couldn't remember which aisle she had already traveled or which aisle she had yet to visit. Embarrassed by this odd sensation, she said nothing to her friend and tried to act normal. Then Norma asked her to check the price of a table that they had both admired a few minutes before. Jill willed herself to comply with this request, but she didn't know which way to walk to find the table. Like Alice in Wonderland, she found that everywhere she turned was the opposite of where she wanted to go. In a stupor, she wandered through the store. She felt frustrated and helpless, but afraid of looking foolish, she didn't ask for help. Finally she stood still and concentrated on the table, determined to move the right way. But still she couldn't force herself to figure it out.

A few weeks later, she had a similarly jarring experience of spatial disorientation. One evening, she and Norma met after work to drive around the city in search of a larger apartment. As they approached a familiar intersection, Jill realized that she didn't know which way to turn. She knew these streets well; she had driven through this intersection hundreds of times before. But now—like Charlie, who in a dreamy state doesn't know how to get home—Jill had no idea where to go.

As before, she said nothing to Norma. Instead, she slowed the car to a stop and shifted into neutral. Norma looked at her and asked what on earth she was doing. Jill could not respond. She vaguely sensed that she had done something wrong. Finally she admitted, "I don't know which way to go."

Norma, recalling her absentmindedness in the furniture store, said, "You know, Jill, your memory has been really screwy for a while."

It was true. From time to time Jill's memory had been impaired by TLE seizures in the part of her brain that controls her sense of where she is in space. As a result, she had dreamy

states in which familiar places, like the store and the intersection, seemed strange. This kind of state—called a *jamais vu,* the
French for "never seen before"—is the opposite of the *déjà vu*
experienced by Penfield's patients in Montreal. At the time, however, Jill knew nothing of TLE or the seizure activity in her brain.
In response, she ignored the odd new sensations, denied them,
or blamed them on stress and lack of sleep.

Several weeks later, she began having difficulty remembering familiar words, names, and numbers. Now and then she
recalled the digits of her own telephone number out of
sequence, in the same way that Dostoevsky during seizures forgot the names or faces of family and friends. At times she could
not connect her thoughts with words—"an awful feeling."
These memory problems rapidly changed Jill's life. She gave up
her daily habit of doing the *New York Times* crossword puzzle.
Her finances, always disorganized, now unraveled. She mis-
placed money, sometimes hundreds of dollars at a time, and
she frequently lost bills. Dunning notices arrived, but she didn't
see them, because she had begun throwing all her mail,
unopened, in a drawer. Eventually the city immobilized her car
because of the $520 she owed in parking tickets, the electric
company shut off her power until she paid her outstanding
bills, and an IRS collector demanded immediate payment of
long overdue taxes. "I've always been bad, but now I'm the
worst money manager I know," Jill lamented. Although she
earned a salary of more than seventy thousand dollars a year,
Ted observed, "she had trouble with the basic elements of her
personal life, such as handling money and keeping good credit.
Lately, she's had a lot of bad luck; it seems there's a new
episode every week." Within a few months, she was mugged,
robbed twice, and had her car broken into. These setbacks only
made her more anxious, which intensified her forgetfulness,
increasing her "bad luck."

In the meantime, her emotions began to change, as a result
of still undetected events in the emotional region of her brain.
She noticed that her feelings—especially her negative feelings—
seemed to intensify. Jill, a self-described "people person" who
establishes rapport easily, had always been rich in feeling, but
now she was more "mercurial" than ever before. She occasionally experienced a powerful euphoria that she could not explain,

and she often fell into extremely dark moods of anger or depression.

Alongside these emotional changes came physical problems. Now and then she felt stirrings of nausea in her stomach. She had dizzy spells and occasionally passed out. On a weekend getaway with friends in the country, her legs "turned to Jell-O" when the blast of heat from an opened oven reduced the oxygen to her brain, causing her to fall down. Another day, while climbing a long flight of stairs at an antiques store, she became so dizzy that she nearly fell. She developed piercing headaches and intermittent pain in her eyes—"as if they're whirling around, not totally wired into my brain." Even her appearance changed: friends occasionally saw a kind of shadow come over her usually bright face.

Oddest of Jill's undiagnosed symptoms were her "funny smells." Several months after the first attacks of *jamais vu*, she began having brief, pungent hallucinations of rotten tuna fish, rancid garlic, or "dead mouse." Sometimes the smell was of celery, so intense that she had the unpleasant sensation of "drowning in a sea of celery," a vegetable that she ordinarily likes. These hallucinations were more or less disturbing, depending on where and how relaxed she was. If she smelled tuna during her morning shower, she could ignore it and finish washing her hair. At work, though, the smells were disruptive. When she smelled garlic during a presentation to the board, she became nervous and confused. She sniffed the air. If she was lucky, Ted or one of her subordinates would sense her distress, step in, and take over the presentation.

These smells proved to be the clue to her diagnosis in the summer of 1984, by which time she had lived with seizures for roughly a year. During that year, she had described her symptoms to several doctors, including her internist and the psychotherapist whom she had been seeing since the difficult end in early 1983 of a long-distance relationship with a German entrepreneur fifteen years her senior. The doctors, not knowing what was wrong with her, had referred her to a neurologist at Beth Israel Hospital, where Norman Geschwind was chief. The neurologist, Michael Ronthal, was stumped by her complaints until Jill mentioned her funny smells, which made him think of TLE. Olfactory hallucinations—a common seizure state—result

from epileptic discharge in the olfactory region, near the temporal lobes. Ronthal realized at once that TLE could also explain
Jill's many other complaints—intermittent gastrointestinal pain,
intense emotions, spatial disorientation, and forgetfulness. He
immediately questioned her about the smells, to determine if
they were consistent with olfactory hallucinations, which tend to
be brief and unsavory. "How long do your smells last?"

"A minute or two."

"Are any of them pleasant?"

"No."

Based on her answers, he told her that he thought she had
seizures. Like the doctor who first suspected Charlie's TLE, he
did not say "epilepsy," a word that he thought would frighten Jill.
Such caution is widespread. A recent edition of a standard neurology textbook advises that the word *epilepsy*, although "a useful medical term, . . . still has unpleasant connotations and is
probably best avoided . . . with patients, until . . . the . . . public
be-comes more enlightened."

"What do you mean, seizures?" Jill asked Ronthal.

"Oh, well," he replied, "you have these electrical impulses in
your brain that are charging and misfiring and not connecting
and all going off at the wrong time."

"What does *that* mean?"

"We have to do an EEG." He said to return to the hospital for
the test in seven weeks. Two weeks later, when she passed out
again, this time at work, she called Ronthal, who said to take a
taxi to the emergency room. Upon her arrival, he was not there.
A resident in neurology read what Ronthal had written on her
chart and gave her a prescription for Dilantin, 300 milligrams
that night and 300 milligrams more the next morning. Jill asked
the resident what the drug was for.

"It's for seizures," he said, avoiding both the charged word
epilepsy and the accurate word *anticonvulsant*.

Dazed and disoriented, Jill went home, took the pills, and
went to sleep. The drug affected her dramatically: the next morning she was so dizzy she couldn't walk. She called Ronthal, who
said, "Oh yes, it may make you feel confused and dizzy. Take
three hundred milligrams more." During her entire first week on
Dilantin, the drug kept her from going to work.

In the meantime, Ronthal pushed up the schedule for her

EEG. When she had the test, the technician used "sphenoidal" electrodes, which are inserted through the skin of the upper cheek and the place where the jawbones meet in order to rest close to the temporal lobes, increasing the chance of detecting abnormalities there. The next day, she called Ronthal's office for the results. The doctor's secretary said he was busy. When Jill explained who she was and why she had called, the secretary said, "The test came back positive." Jill asked what that meant. The secretary said, "You have epilepsy."

"What?" Jill exclaimed, horrified by the word, as the doctor had predicted. Unlike those patients who feel that naming epilepsy makes it easier to live with by establishing the reality of their strange symptoms, Jill wishes that she had never been told of her disorder. The diagnosis came like a verdict of guilty. "It was like having somebody whack me on the head a few times and say, 'Now you've got *this*!' Having a name attached to it makes it seem more serious, especially since epilepsy is a very taboo disease."

The diagnosis was a turning point for Jill. Unlike Charlie, whose life returned nearly to normal once he was stabilized on anticonvulsant drugs, Jill has been permanently changed by TLE. "It has been really hard for me to adjust," she said. "It was like one day I was somewhat all right, and the next day I just went down the tubes." TLE, which directly affects her brain, the organ containing her sense of self, has cost her a sense of security and personal control. "Having TLE is very different from having, say, an abscess on my arm; then I could just cut my arm off. TLE invades your *self*, it screws around with your personality, and it comes through in how you function. Oh, I can still do a tough job; I buck up. But I'm significantly changed as a person and in how I view myself and the world." She no longer feels confident that she can moderate her own emotions, behavior, and thoughts, being ever at the mercy of the next seizure. "Emotionally or physically, I'm not the same person I was before. And I can't go back. That's probably the toughest thing. I've had to leave a part of myself behind."

Along with the diagnosis came unpleasant questions about the cause of her TLE. Donald Schomer, the Beth Israel neurologist who took on her case after Ronthal made the diagnosis, quickly ascertained that, like Charlie, she had none of the obvious causes of epilepsy, such as birth trauma or head injury. Since adult-onset seizures suggested the possibility of a tumor, Schomer recommended that Jill have brain scans, which showed no evidence of a tumor. According to the doctor, the only suggestive or relevant episode in her history occurred before she was born. Following her parents' marriage, in 1945, her mother had four pregnancies, all miscarriages. In 1949, a doctor prescribed to her mother the antimiscarriage drug diethylstilbestrol, or DES; the next year, she gave birth to a son. Two years later, while pregnant with Jill, the mother again took DES. Although Jill seemed perfectly healthy from birth until the start of her seizures, Schomer suspected that the DES had caused her brain to develop slightly abnormally in the womb. The resulting physical abnormality, which he thought was in her hypothalamus, a structure deep in the temporal lobe that regulates hormone function through the pituitary gland, could alter electrical activity in her brain, causing seizures.

Many of the offspring of women who used DES have serious medical problems, and the drug has long been banned. Among the daughters of DES users, according to Schomer, there are unusually high rates of temporal lobe dysfunction, which can include TLE, vaginal cancer, ovarian cysts, and fertility problems. In the months following Jill's diagnosis she learned that she had all these problems except the cancer: hormonal tests showed that she does not ovulate; and a gynecologist found ovarian cysts. "Every time I go to the doctor something else isn't working," she complained to Schomer. "My body is going weird on me."

Her seizures worsened soon after her diagnosis, despite treatment with various anticonvulsants, and they increasingly interfered with her work. Job stress increased their frequency, while the seizures in turn increased the stress she felt at the office. She had terrible headaches, often lasting all day, during which she couldn't concentrate. She sat through interviews and meetings unable to focus her mind. Her moods fluctuated wildly. Her feelings seemed entirely out of control. "If I feel really bad for several days, I get really depressed," she said, "because I think that I'll never stop feeling this way." She became more forgetful. After a meeting of the company's board of directors at which all parties agreed on a percentage figure for a raise that would be given to every employee, she left to compute the actual cost of the raise. When she presented her calculations at the next meeting, everyone present was amazed: she had used the wrong figure. Before, she had always been able to rely on her excellent memory for numbers. Horrified by this mistake and unable to stop her seizures, she began taking extensive notes at work.

In time, it seemed that all she could do was to keep up with her job, and even that often felt like too much. The only time since her diagnosis when she had consistently felt well was during a three-month medical leave from work in 1986. Feeling like "a wreck" when the leave started, she improved dramatically over the course of the three months spent relaxing. Within weeks of returning to work, though, she was as tired and stressed as before. Aware that she could not justify regular three-month leaves, she fantasized about quitting her job. She imagined giving the company president a month's notice and dropping out of the corporate rat race for six months to a year in order to travel to the Far East. Yet she knew this was impractical: she had little money saved, and her job provided financial security and health insurance.

Still, the idea of quitting kept coming up. Waiting in line to buy hot dogs at a Fenway Park concession stand during a baseball game one summer evening about five years after her diagnosis, she heard the teenage vendor yell, "NO MORE PRETZELS!" Jill's face lit up. "No more pretzels!" she repeated, enthralled. "I love it!" She wished she could use a line like that at work. "NO MORE JOBS!" she cried to an imaginary corps of interviewees. "We're closed!"

Seizure-based changes made her feel that her once-varied options in life were falling away. TLE affected her personal life, reducing her chances, she thought, of marrying and having a family. During her twenties, while concentrating on building a career, she had dated numerous men, living with one boyfriend for two years. When she developed TLE at thirty-one, she was dating casually and still smarting from the end of the relationship with the German man. After her diagnosis, her caution about getting deeply involved with men increased. Her mother, who was eager for Jill to marry, lamented the sudden change: "Jill always had a boyfriend from the time she was twelve, but lately things have kind of leveled off, and she doesn't have someone consistently anymore. I don't know what's happened." One factor, according to Jill, was her new knowledge that she would have difficulty becoming pregnant: she would have to take a fertility drug in order to ovulate; and she would have to stop taking anticonvulsants, which are known to cause birth defects. Moreover, she felt uncomfortable telling men she dated about her TLE. Most people have never heard of it. When she had to cancel engagements at the last minute because of seizures, she felt she couldn't say why. "I have to be careful what I say, because many people are ignorant about epilepsy: they expect me to be insane or totally unstable." As a result of these fears, she said, "My sex life is nonexistent lately; I've dated hardly at all."

The few men she did fall for in the years following her diagnosis were not eligible, not available, or not around. "She likes men who don't adore her and who aren't willing to make commitments," her colleague Ted said. Paul Spiers, a young neuropsychologist who began giving her psychotherapy after her diagnosis, replacing the first psychiatrist, said, "TLE makes her not want to socialize because she never knows when she'll have a spell; it makes her feel she's not attractive to the opposite sex; and it makes her not want to take risks. Jill had a normal life for thirty years, and it's hard for her to accept her epilepsy. It doesn't mesh with her self-image to see herself as damaged or impaired."

In response to the diagnosis, she isolated herself, accepting little support from anyone except medical personnel. At work, she let her frequent absences go unexplained. A private person, she felt uncomfortable sharing her experiences even with friends. Rather than risk rejection or embarrassment, she refused to make dates or, if friends forced them on her, canceled at the last minute or simply failed to show up. She unplugged her phone machine and sometimes her phone. She disliked offending people, but felt she had no choice. "I want to be by myself," she said. "I don't want to talk about TLE." Her family provided little help. She was not close with her brother, who lived on the West Coast. Her father, a retired businessman, was coping with cancer at the time of her diagnosis, leaving him little energy or time for Jill. Her mother, a fashion consultant, might have supported her during her adjustment to TLE, except that she took an even more skeptical stance toward the diagnosis than did Ted. The mother, a powerful figure who had always told Jill that nothing was more fulfilling than being a wife and mother, refused to believe that her daughter has epilepsy; she considered the diagnosis an "excuse" for not finding a husband. Before long, it seemed, Jill's three professional caretakers—the neurologist; a nurse who specializes in epilepsy; and the new psychotherapist—had become a substitute family. She saw one or two of them every month, and increasingly viewed them as her primary sources of support.

According to these caretakers, TLE limited the scope of Jill's life but it did not bring on a clear case of Geschwind's syndrome. The traits in her were subtle, neither prominent nor disabling. Because of the early damage to her brain, she may have had several of the traits even before developing seizures. According to Spiers, she gives evidence of "some circumstantiality [an inordinate attention to detail that is akin to hypergraphia] and some of the temper, and she's probably hyposexual, on and off." Schomer added that certain "personality issues make her fit into what we see with TLE. She may be hyposexual—her relationships with men are superficial—and she started out philosophical, with an unusual, lifelong interest in philosophy." In college she majored in philosophy, writing her thesis on the religious ethic in the work of Dostoevsky, of whose epilepsy she was unaware.

Schomer expressed private concerns that if Jill's seizures continue unabated she could gradually undergo a long-term personality change involving an intensification of Geschwind's syndrome and sometimes including psychotic behavior. This happens in 15 percent of longtime TLE patients roughly fourteen years after the onset of seizures, perhaps because recurring seizures can permanently alter emotional areas of the brain. According to David Bear, a psychiatrist, the psychosis seen with TLE is not true schizophrenia but rather "schizophreniform," or schizophreniclike, because the patient, unlike a schizophrenic, maintains "strong affect" and a "high level of interpersonal functioning." To determine whether a long-term personality change occurs in Jill, Schomer hopes to examine her in ten or twenty years, noting in particular if her pre-existing traits intensify.

Chances are, Spiers concurred, Jill will gradually become more religious, more aggressive, and even less interested in sex.

Despite these real and potential difficulties, TLE brought an unexpected benefit: occasional dreamy states consisting of sensory hallucinations that Jill adores. She fades out, feeling pleasantly disconnected from the world around her, disembodied, weightless, or as if she were invisible. Sometimes she has out-of-body experiences in which she feels herself split: her mind seems to break away and hover several feet above her body, giving her the sensation of "watching myself." At other times, she feels she is floating. People who are with her during these enjoyable seizures notice little change in her appearance except that she looks dazed, "out of it," in another world, for a moment or two. During a conversation, Jill may fall silent for twenty seconds, return to normal consciousness, and then say, vaguely, "Oh, did you ask me something?" These "nice" seizures, like the others, are beyond her control. "You don't say, 'I'm going to check out.' It just happens to you."

Jill also developed visual hallucinations, which are caused by epileptic discharge spreading to the part of the brain that controls vision, behind the temporal lobes. Stationary objects, such as a chair or a table, sometimes appear to shrink or to expand, common seizure states that are known, respectively, as micropsia and macropsia. These sensations frighten her, but all of her other seizural visions are pleasant. She frequently has the feeling that all the colors in the world around her are unusually brilliant and mesmerizing, a feeling that makes her euphoric. "It's a wonderfully altered state of consciousness," she said, "like stepping into another dimension that doesn't really exist—but it does exist, in your mind!" Patients with similar seizures report visions of flashing "Christmas lights." In still other visual seizures, Jill sees a spot of beautiful blue in the top right corner of her visual field, which she finds "nice, creative, calming." The first time she saw this, it was night and she was driving. In the darkness, the blue spot looked like a beacon. Suspecting that it was a seizure, Jill carefully drove home.

These pleasurable mental states have given Jill a new perspective on the mind, "a view of the world other people don't get." She explained, "TLE has made me realize there's a whole other realm out there that, although it may be bad, is fascinating. My nice seizures—the colors and floating sensations—are the closest to religious or spiritual feelings that I've ever had, and they've made me understand for the first time how people can think they've discovered God." Jill is not religious, but these seizural feelings helped her to understand why some cultures revered epilepsy and considered epileptics the recipients of spiritual knowledge. "Although epilepsy makes people uncomfortable, it's also a plus: TLE makes you see the quirks of the brain, its mystery. You can't see or touch the brain; you can't get hold of it. You know nothing about it, except that it's supposed to work. Most people think of their brain only as intellect, as opposed to how they see, smell, and taste. When I have these wonderful states of feeling I'm somewhere else, I'm fascinated!" She longed to find some way of expressing these feelings to others, perhaps through writing or art. But the disorder was hard to explain. When she occasionally described her symptoms to friends, they reacted with surprise and concern. Disconcerted by this, Jill kept most of her seizural feelings to herself.

Others may have used seizures similar to Jill's as the basis for constructing imaginary worlds. The eighteenth-century Anglo-Irish clergyman and satirist Jonathan Swift is now thought to have had epilepsy. The miniature and mammoth peoples, Lilliputians and Brobdingnagians, whom Gulliver encounters in his travels suggest that Swift experienced micropsia and macropsia during seizures. In the nineteenth century, while van Gogh and Dostoevsky were transforming their experiences of epilepsy into drawings and novels, another writer invented a character whose bizarre adventures are now thought to be fictionalized accounts of seizures. In *Alice's Adventures in Wonderland* and *Through the Looking-Glass*, according to Paul Spiers, "Lewis Carroll was probably writing about his own temporal lobe seizures."

To Spiers, many of the experiences of the child heroine Alice sound like TLE seizures, some of them similar to Jill's. The very sensation initiating Alice's adventures—that of falling down a hole—is described in seizures by people with TLE. Like Jill and Gulliver, Alice often feels that objects are shrinking or expanding before her eyes; her own body contracts to a height of ten inches and then grows to a height of nine feet. A contemporary of Jill's who has experienced this kind of seizure described feeling his body expanding to exactly one and one-sixteenth its usual size, causing him to fear that his personality might enter the sixteenth part and separate permanently from the rest; during the seizure he could hear himself saying, "Yes, please," but he felt that the person speaking was not he.

Alice and Jill share other seizure states. Alice has frequent attacks of *jamais vu*, which make her spatially insecure, and she has sudden, unprompted changes in emotion, such as bursts of tears, panic, or rage. Like Jill, she also experiences wonderful states of being. "I feel somehow as if I was getting invisible," Alice exclaims. In Looking-Glass Land she "ran down stairs—or, at least, it wasn't exactly running, but a new invention for getting down stairs quickly and easily/. . . She just kept the tips of her fingers on the hand-rail, and floated gently down without even touching the stairs with her feet: then she floated on through the hall, and would have gone straight out at the door in the same way, if she hadn't caught hold of the doorpost. She was getting a little giddy with so much floating in the air." When Lewis Carroll wrote these accounts in his thirties, apparently neither he nor his doctors were aware of his disorder. Not until twenty years later did both he and his doctors conclude that he suffered from epilepsy.

"I had an attack ('epileptiform' Dr. Morshead called it) which left me with a sort of headache and not feeling my usual self for a week or ten days," the fifty-four-year-old Charles Lutwidge Dodgson, who used Lewis Carroll as a *nom de plume*, wrote in his diary on January 20, 1886. Morshead used the term *epileptiform*, or epilepticlike, to indicate that Dodgson's seizure was not the well-known grand mal type. When the doctor asked if Dodgson knew of any epilepsy in his family, he said no. Yet he had prematurely white hair, which is common in families with epilepsy, and he displayed physical signs of neurological damage from childhood, including deafness in one ear and a stammer. Dodgson also had a strikingly asymmetrical face, which, like Charlie's asymmetrical reflexes, often indicates damage to one side of the brain. An acquaintance reported that Dodgson had "two very different profiles; the shape of the eyes [and] the corners of the mouth did not tally." He complained of difficulties eating, relaxing, and sleeping, and he periodically suffered tormenting headaches and visual hallucinations.

Five years later, Dodgson had another seizure, and another

doctor confirmed the diagnosis. This seizure occurred in the chapel at Oxford, the university where he spent most of his life, studying and then lecturing in mathematics. While kneeling in prayer in his pew following the morning service, Dodgson felt a dreamy sensation and fainted, falling to the stone floor of the empty church. He lay unconscious for an hour or so, either because the seizure activity had generalized, causing a secondary grand mal attack, or because he had suffered a concussion when he fell. Eventually he awoke from "an uneasy dream" to find his shirt and face bloody. Describing the sensation later to a child, he wrote of thinking to himself "how *very* uncomfortable the pillow is!" For several minutes he felt he was "*still* dreaming," and as in the earlier seizure he had a headache, this one lasting nearly a week. The symptoms and the prolonged headache, which often follows a TLE seizure, convinced his doctor that the attack was epileptic. Mistakenly thinking that seizures are seasonal, the doctor advised him not to exhaust himself by traveling in the winter, the time of year when both his "epileptic attacks," as the doctor put it, had occurred. Following this advice, Dodgson stayed home the next Christmas, spending the holiday alone in his apartment above an Oxford library.

In personality, too, the solitary writer was typical of people with TLE. According to Spiers, Dodgson possessed an undisputed case of Geschwind's syndrome, the group of characteristics that some doctors now use as a diagnostic aid. His hypergraphia was astounding. At age thirteen, he single-handedly produced a magazine containing fifteen verses and twenty-eight pages of sketches and watercolors. As an adult he wrote compulsively, publishing numerous pamphlets and books of poetry, mathematics, logic, drawings, and fantasy, and keeping a daily journal for more than four decades. A prodigious correspondent, he penned roughly two thousand letters a year. The meticulous twenty-four-volume log he kept of every letter he received or sent, from his late twenties until his death at age sixty-five, contains 98,721 entries. A third of his life went to receiving letters, he once said, and the other two-thirds to writing them. His texts, like those of Waxman and Geschwind's hypergraphic patients, displayed quirks characteristic of the syndrome: mirror writing, extensive annotation, numerous drawings in the borders, and almost exclusive reliance on purple ink. According to the literary critic V. S. Pritchett, Dodgson was "married to his inkpot and a harem of ingenious pens of his own invention."

Other traits of Geschwind's syndrome fueled this hypergraphia. A devout Protestant who, like Jonathan Swift, was an ordained minister, Dodgson composed many sermons and religious tracts. Prudish and fastidious in matters of etiquette, he had a temper when offended; poor manners, cricket playing on Sundays, and incorrect grammar drove him wild. According to an Oxford associate, he was "the most prolific malcontent," sending letters to the university administration "calling attention to, or asking for the redress of miscellaneous grievances: The messengers sometimes clear the letter-boxes two minutes before the stated hour. . . . There is a 'dangerous effluvium caused by some defect of drainage' which makes the New Common Room 'quite uninhabitable'. . . . He requires an electric bell-push in each of his two bedrooms. Please tell the kitchen to send him *no more smoked ham.* . . . And so on; and so on. . . ."

In relationships, Dodgson was both sticky and asexual. He lived alone, never married, and apparently never experienced sex with another person. His prized companions over the decades were prepubescent girls. He lavished attention on scores of them, sending them adoring notes and begging them to visit him. In his bachelor rooms, he plied the girls with tea and cakes, sometimes paid them to stay longer than they wanted, and frequently photographed them in costumes or in the nude. Evidently neither the children he befriended nor their parents ever questioned the motives of this timid, gentle, stuttering Oxford don.

The Reverend Dodgson's unusual behavior did not trouble either his contemporaries, who trusted and admired him, or the generations of children who have adored his books of fantasy since his death. In Lewis Carroll, as in Dostoevsky, Geschwind's syndrome had distinct benefits: in the constrained world of the perfect Victorian gentleman such traits as hypergraphia, stickiness, extreme religiosity, fussiness, and altered sexuality all had their place. In a different person, time, and place, however, the characteristics that mingled in Lewis Carroll can be extremely difficult to live with. Either because the person is less able to adapt to them or because the traits appear in even brighter hues,

Geschwind's syndrome can lead to socially unacceptable behavior, to the appearance of psychiatric disease, and even to criminal acts.

In a classroom in one of the white marble Greco-Roman halls defining the central quadrangle of Harvard Medical School, Gloria Johnson sat quietly awaiting her introduction to an audience of aspiring physicians. She had been invited by her doctor, David Bear, to be a "guest lecturer" with him when he visited this spring-semester course in neurosciences. Gloria, a small, middle-aged woman with a smooth baby face, had dressed for the occasion in bright new sneakers, a red-and-white polka-dotted dress, and a white blazer; matching red barrettes held back her short hair. The lapel button announcing her as a Famous Person was a gift from Bear that he had pinned on her just before the class. He had told her that he wanted her to share with medical students her experience of TLE. He had told his students that she is a remarkable example of a medical syndrome demonstrating the effects of seizures on the emotional parts of the brain.

The physical bases of human emotions was Bear's subject for the day. "I'm a psychiatrist, so I'm interested in emotion," he noted with a smile. A tall, lean man in his forties with bushy, salt-and-pepper hair, Bear had studied science and medicine at Harvard, had done an internship in neurology under Geschwind, and was now on staff at hospitals affiliated with Harvard Medical School. He told the class that the common emotions, which he called "feeling states related to biological drives," are anger, fear, hunger, and sexual yearning. This quartet, he added, "is sometimes called the four F's: fight, flight, feeding, and . . . sex." At this, several of his students grinned, but Gloria's somber expression remained. She felt apprehensive about the remarks she had been asked to make. And, herself of African descent, she was troubled that there was not one person of color among the twenty or so medical students in the room.

Since emotions occur in both humans and animals, Bear continued, Charles Darwin considered them essential for species' survival. Animals and humans express emotions somewhat differently: animal emotion seems largely automatic, while the control of emotion in humans is subtle and complex; and the range of human emotion is far more varied than that in animals, contributing to religion, language, and art. In both animals and humans, however, emotions are governed and regulated by electrical activity in a region near the center of the brain, part of the temporal lobe. In animals, the removal of this brain region causes dramatic emotional changes: cats become extremely aggressive and sexually indiscriminate; monkeys become docile and unafraid. Although surgical experimentation on humans is not allowed, Bear said, "we do have the example of temporal lobe epilepsy, the most common of the adult epilepsies," which shows us the function of this part of the brain. While TLE seizures are "overwhelmingly unemotional" in content, he added, the continuous abnormal brain activity underlying them can alter overall emotional function, making people more or less angry, or more or less interested in sex. "If repeated seizures damage the brain at the level of the circuitry that tells us if a certain emotion is socially appropriate—how angry you can be at your boss, or whether or not you ought to reach over and wolf down somebody else's food—this can cause emotional problems.

"Now Mrs. Johnson here," he continued, gesturing toward Gloria, "has had temporal lobe epilepsy nearly all her life." Hearing her name, Gloria turned expectantly to face the class. She listened carefully as Bear sketched the outlines of her medical history, her bulging, watery eyes making her seem constantly on the verge of tears. Born in Boston in 1930 to recent immigrants from the West Indies, Gloria, like van Gogh, had a difficult birth. The umbilical cord was wrapped around her neck, cutting off her oxygen, which, Bear thought, probably caused part of her brain to scar. Although her TLE was not diagnosed until she was thirty-seven, her earliest seizures—staring spells, lapses in normal consciousness and memory, and isolated bodily convulsions—started when she was only one or two years old. She wet her bed until she was thirteen, probably, he said, because of night seizures in which her sphincter muscles relaxed. She dropped out of high school at fourteen, worked briefly as a stitcher in a factory, and got a job dancing at night clubs. In her twenties, as her dancing career wound down, she trained at a cosmetology school to become a hairdresser; within several years, she had become an instructor.

Gloria's undiagnosed seizures continued throughout her adolescence and early adulthood. She had severe headaches in the back of one side of her head, during which the eye on that side wandered and she sometimes passed out. She developed spells in which she thought she was spinning around, she was nauseated, she felt hot, her vision blurred or doubled, and she seemed to be choking. Now and then she heard male voices mumbling, some telling her that she had "better die." At other times she heard the distant sound of a telephone ringing, or a knocking that seemed so real she would answer her door, only to find no one there. She had difficulty sleeping, probably because of night seizures. She had dramatic mood swings, going from rage to deep depression. She experienced agonizing waves of dread, similar to Jill's panic attacks, in which she felt certain that "something very bad is going to happen to me."

In her late twenties, these problems became more frequent and intense, so that Gloria was having between sixty and one hundred seizures of one kind or another every day. She responded by drinking heavily, behavior that recalls van Gogh's. As in many epileptics, alcohol only made her symptoms worse. In despair borne of seizures, when even death seemed preferable to her psychic pain, she repeatedly overdosed on sleeping pills or other medications that her doctors had prescribed for depression or psychosis. After each suicide attempt, she spent a week or more as a psychiatric inpatient at a state mental hospital or at Boston City Hospital, where in the decade prior to her diagnosis she spent the equivalent of more than two years.

The doctors who saw Gloria over that decade diagnosed her as having myriad psychiatric disorders, including "paranoid schizophrenia," "depressive psychosis," "hysterical personality disorder," and "psychoneurotic depressive reaction associated with anxiety and long-standing problems of homosexual orientation." Bear would later refute all these psychiatric labels, saying that Gloria had neither a personality disorder nor a psychosis: "She's tempestuous and paranoid to start [with], but her long-range judgment is preserved." The numerous antipsychotic drugs, such as Mellaril and Thorazine, and antidepressants that doctors gave her in the 1960s had no beneficial effect, and the antipsychotics actually intensified her seizures. This is a common reaction of TLE patients to these drugs, and it is now considered a clue that a patient has epilepsy rather than a psychiatric disease.

Moreover, Gloria had none of the mental deterioration common in psychosis. A doctor who saw her when she was thirty-four observed "no abnormalities . . . in orientation, memory, attention, concentration, . . . and intelligence. Her insight and judgment are not impaired. . . . No delusions or misinterpretations. . . . Very frequently patient thinks that 'everybody is picking on me,' either because she is a Negro or because of other real or imaginary reasons. . . . But very soon she is able to see the real reasons for things." Despite her sanity, doctors who saw her during these years did not suspect epilepsy. In 1964, when Gloria was thirty-three, one doctor went so far as to state that she "has no neurological disease," providing what Bear later called "not a very thoughtful analysis, even then."

But some doctor must have suspected neurological damage, because starting at age thirty-four Gloria was given occasional EEGs. The results of these tests were mostly normal, as is common in known cases of TLE: an ordinary EEG with ordinary electrodes often fails to detect epileptic discharge in the temporal lobes, which are deep in the brain. However, when Gloria was thirty-six, two EEGs with ordinary electrodes revealed electrical abnormalities in the top and front of her left temporal lobe. Subsequent EEGs, some with depth electrodes that were surgically implanted in her brain, consistently showed abnormalities in her right temporal lobe. Her "impulsive behavior," a doctor finally wrote in 1967, "may be attributable to organ lesion," or a scar on her brain, which also appeared to cause "temporal lobe seizures."

Gloria had a mixed reaction to the new diagnosis of TLE. She was relieved that her doctors had abandoned psychiatric labels for her problems. Yet she considered epilepsy a serious and frightening disorder. As her doctors prescribed, she began taking the anticonvulsants Mysoline and Dilantin, but these drugs had scant effect on either the frequency or the intensity of her seizures. Like Jill and two-thirds of all TLE patients, she felt that her seizures did not respond well to drugs.

At the time of her visit to Harvard Medical School, she was still taking Dilantin and another anticonvulsant, and still having between ten and fifty seizures daily, far more per day than Charlie or Jill ever had. Gloria's typical seizure, Bear told his students, begins with an unpleasant smell lasting a minute or two. "It's a horrible stink," Gloria interposed, "of feces, urine, or burning kerosene. It's *not* Chanel Number Five." Next she has an automatism, mechanically turning her head or smacking her lips. Her left arm and the left side of her face twitch. From this point on in a seizure, she is not fully aware of what she is doing, and she will not recall her actions later. When asked where she is or what day or month it is, she cannot say for sure. She stares blankly, sometimes for as long as fifteen minutes. Like Dostoevsky, she has bursts of intense emotion—anger, sadness, or fear. Sometimes she loses consciousness and falls down in a grand mal seizure, the result of epileptic activity spreading throughout her brain.

"Now let's talk about your emotions," Bear said to Gloria, nodding his encouragement.

"I've got *strong* emotions," she affirmed with a vigor that made her words seem rehearsed, which, in a sense, they were. Gloria had participated in this lecture with Bear each spring for five years, so she knew what questions to expect. "I'm ready every minute to cut you down!" she warned, glaring at her audience. Like a schoolteacher ensuring that every child is paying attention, she scanned the room. "I don't play," she said. "A person has to be real soft to me or kind. You don't jump at me or bother me, because it's danger on your hands." The students, sitting in rows and listening quietly, did not react. They were accustomed to seeing patients presented by professors as examples of medical conditions. Moreover, Gloria appeared unable to act upon her threat. She sat in a wheelchair, protective cloth braces encasing her ankles, wrists, and neck, all the result of rheumatoid arthritis, a crippling autoimmune disorder, which she developed in her early forties. For unknown reasons, autoimmune disorders occur with unusual frequency in families with epilepsy. Gloria's combined arthritis and TLE led to her early retirement from hairdressing; she now received monthly social security disability and social security insurance payments, food stamps, and fuel assistance from the government.

Staying with her aggression, Bear made what he knew was a vast understatement. "Mrs. Johnson can get quite irritable."

"That's right, Dr. Bear!" she agreed. The students chuckled, not sure what more to expect.

"Has this tendency of yours gotten you into trouble?" the doctor prompted.

"I cut my first husband!" she replied with apparent pride. Gloria was referring to one of the many violent acts that are described, usually with minimal detail or explanation, in her vast medical record. The size of a medical file is one index of a patient's need for care: Gloria's massive file, its many volumes gathered during scores of psychiatric and neurological admissions to Boston hospitals over four decades, is five times the size of Jill's and at least fifty times thicker than the slender file in the office of Charlie's neurologist. In the instance of violence that Gloria mentioned, she was nineteen, living with her first husband, a short-order cook turned soldier, on an army base in Tennessee. In a purported attempt to kill him, she slashed his back with a razor. "He was a bad man," she said later by way of explanation. He recovered from the wound, they lived together "on and off" for the next ten years, and then they were divorced.

Bear glanced down at a page of her medical file, one of several that he had culled and brought with him to the lecture, and asked, "You went to jail?"

"Yeah," she murmured. Convicted in 1949 for the assault on her husband, she had spent several months in a federal prison. While she readily admits her history of violence, she is unwilling to give people who question her many details, fearing that they will think ill of her.

Aware of her need for limits, Bear moved on to another incident. He found the reference in her medical file to the time in her twenties when she beat a policeman unconscious outside a Boston nightclub. "Now, Mrs. Johnson, did you ever attack a policeman?"

"Oh, yeah," she said, with renewed intensity. There were a number of raised eyebrows in the room. It was hard to believe that this engaging little woman could have done such violent deeds. Yet Gloria, unlike Charlie and Jill, has had problems with aggression all her life. In a family of ten children, she stood out as "the bad one," irritable, always ready to fight. "I just couldn't obey," she once told Bear. "I couldn't behave. I felt I always had to protect myself. I used to beat the other children." A doctor reported that as a child Gloria tried to kill her father with a knife. In her twenties she spent a week in an army hospital in

Kentucky "for aggression" of unspecified particulars. In her early thirties she tried to castrate an unsatisfactory sexual partner with a broken bottle. "She partly succeeded," a doctor noted, without elaborating. While a psychiatric inpatient at Boston City Hospital in the 1960s, she was "abusive and assaultive" to other patients and to attendants. Summing up her character, Vernon Mark, a neurosurgeon who knew her for twenty years, stated bluntly, "She has a killer personality. She never actually killed anyone, but the difference between killing and maiming is luck."

"Are you ever angry at politicians?" Bear asked her, hoping she would talk about her extraordinary, pervasive anger at any societal injustice, whether racism, ageism, or sexism.

Gloria didn't realize what Bear was after. "Who?" she said quizzically, looking up at him.

"Are you angry at Reagan, perhaps?" he suggested, referring to the President, then in his second term.

"Oh, Dr. Bear!" she cried, thinking she had caught on. "I *said* you should have let that guy you defended—what was his name? Hinckley!—out of prison." Bear, who frequently testifies in court on behalf of people with neurologic damage who are accused of crimes, had been an expert witness for the defense in the 1982 trial of John Hinckley, Jr., for shooting the President and three other people in 1981. Bear's testimony that Hinckley was psychotic and thus not responsible for his actions was a major factor in the verdict of not guilty by reason of insanity. Gloria sympathized with the defendant, whom she viewed as a victim, and she abhorred the conservative policies of the President. "That man Reagan *should* be shot!" she exclaimed. "He's got Alzheimer's." Some of the students laughed.

Bear decided to leave the subject of aggression and move on to another trait of Geschwind's syndrome. He had hoped to explore Gloria's extreme compassion toward those in trouble, but he could return to that later in the lecture. Rather than exhaustively listing particulars, he wanted to give the students an overall impression of Gloria's character. "Now, Mrs. Johnson," he said, "do people get the feeling that sex is on your mind all the time?"

"Oh, yeah," she said, "since I was three." Unlike Charlie, who says that sex is a subject he prefers not to get into, Gloria is happy to discuss with doctors her rich sexual history. Her medical records are studded with remarks about her sexual behavior, some vague or slightly contradictory, but all confirming her powerful, nearly lifelong interest in sex. According to a medical history taken when she was thirty-four, she began having sexual relations with boys when she was five or six years old, and she found the experience "fascinating." Her heterosexual activity led to numerous pregnancies, all of which ended in abortions. Her homosexual activity began at age seven or eight, with one of her sisters, and continued thereafter; at the time of the history, she spoke of a "steady girlfriend." She masturbated daily from age eleven, the record said, "even if she has normal sex relationships." She "kept up all three lives: 1. masturbation; 2. homosexual; 3. heterosexual experiences until present day." Doctors described her "indiscriminate use of any thing or any body as a source of sexual gratification." At the hospital in an "open ward setting, she was masturbating eighteen to twenty times a day. She had a history of promiscuous sexual relations with lesbian prostitutes; she would also go to bed with two or more men at a time and exhaust them all with her demands."

"Was sex ever part of your livelihood?" Bear asked.

"Oh, yeah," she said casually.

"Your sexual preference?"

"Both ways," she replied. "I like it *every* way." To demonstrate these proclivities, Gloria pointed at the young woman who had accompanied her to the class and said, "That one's got nice hips!" The woman, a nun and parochial-school teacher who visits Gloria from time to time, blushed and lowered her eyes. Gloria turned her sultry gaze on her doctor. "What about *you*, Dr. Bear? You're pretty cute!"

Bear suppressed a grin. In his view, she sometimes exaggerates for effect—as when she told him that she had had sex with dogs—but most of what she says seems true. Long before he described Geschwind's syndrome to her, she displayed the traits in striking array. After their first appointment, on May 4, 1979, he wrote this note: "Patient has many behaviors seen during *interictal* period of TLE," or between seizures. She is "emotional, tearful, extremely aggressive, religious, unusual [in her] sexual orientations, circumstantial, and perseverative," the last quality referring to what Norman Geschwind called stickiness. A few years later, Bear added to that list, describing Gloria as having hypergraphia, irritability, "pansexuality," and a "preoccupation with religious and philosophical matters." It is the unusual intensity of these traits in her, conspiring to make a textbook case of Geschwind's syndrome, that prompted Bear to invite her to join him for this lecture year after year. He considers her not typical of people with TLE, but brilliantly illustrative of the disorder's effect on human emotions. He speculates that the intensity of these traits in her results from brain damage to her prefrontal lobes, a region that moderates the emotions, enabling a person to be discreet and circumspect. This damage could have occurred during her loss of oxygen at birth, after a head injury, or as a result of long-standing seizures, which can alter brain tissue. In Bear's view, Gloria is unlike most TLE patients in that "she doesn't take a moment to think of the consequences before she yields to strong impulses. Most people with TLE have strong feelings—of righteous indignation, say—but they don't express them as flagrantly as Gloria." Her extreme personality is thus the result both of overstimulation of her temporolimbic structures and of reduced inhibition in her frontal lobes. Not only is her emotional volume turned up, but also the mechanism that screens her emotions is out of order. The result is Geschwind's syndrome enhanced.

Turning to the subject of hyperreligiosity, Bear asked Gloria, "How about your religious feelings?"

"Oh, I asked the bishop would he marry me," she replied. She had indeed done so that morning, in a telephone conversation with the Most Reverend Lawrence J. Riley, an auxiliary bishop in the Roman Catholic Archdiocese of Boston. As always when she says outrageous things to him during their frequent conversations, the bishop had laughed, asked her to pray for him, and kindly said he had to go. She calls him several times a month, and he has learned that giving her a few minutes of his time causes less trouble than trying to avoid her calls.

Gloria was raised as a Catholic, and although her arthritis now prevents her from attending services regularly, she remains deeply religious. She prays and reads the Bible daily, recording her spiritual meditations in notebooks and on audio tapes, which she sometimes shares with members of the clergy. She also expresses her religious feelings through the civic activism that she has long considered her work. Troubled by the plight of other elderly, low-income, minority residents of Boston, she spends hours every day phoning the archdiocesan office, public officials at city hall, and Boston journalists to complain about public services, general injustice, social ills, her own suffering, or simply to chat. "I have to help the people who need help," she had told Bear. "City hall hangs up on them; that's not right. But people know the work I do, they call me, I talk with them about their cases, and I go through city hall. I'll keep on calling; no one will shut me up, I don't care *who* it is." On a typical day, she phoned a priest, a nun, seven city hall employees, an editor at the *Boston Herald*, a lawyer who she thought might assist her, and a doctor who she felt had treated her badly. Some of her activism is on her own behalf, such as her successful petition to the city of Boston for a second "handicapped parking" sign outside her house. But many calls are on behalf of others. She demands that city agencies provide social workers and other public assistance to elderly people she knows.

This service extends beyond the poor. "She does favors for her doctors, and she *does* get results," Bear said privately. At one of her appointments, for instance, Bear happened to mention that his wife could not get the gas company to fix their stove in less than a week. "*I* can take care of that," Gloria told him. Later that day she called the gas company repeatedly, demanding that they take care of Bear's stove. Hours later, repairmen appeared at the doctor's house. Similarly, when Gloria's internist complained to her about the huge increase in property taxes on his Boston town house, she took on that problem. She called the assessor's office at city hall again and again until the city agreed to reassess the doctor's property.

Bear cited this behavior as striking evidence of both hyper-religiosity and stickiness. Since her arthritis eliminated most outlets for her anger besides the telephone, her activism also reflects displaced rage. "Her personality problems grow out of sincere feelings of something being wrong," he said. "She is, in her own way, deeply religious, conscientious, and ethical, interested in serving the poor." As Gloria told another doctor, "You don't have to live in a church to be religious."

Moving to yet another trait, Bear asked Gloria if she ever writes. She replied, "Oh, I do that all the time." The doctor riffled through the papers on the desk, found the one he was looking for, and raised a white sheet for the students to see. It was a copy of a page of one of Gloria's journals, in which she records her thoughts, feelings, memories, and lists of information she has gathered over the years, such as all the muscles and bones of the spinal column, which she learned when she took an adult-education course on the human nervous system. Bear included this page in the hypergraphia section of an article about TLE. As he held it aloft, Gloria closed her eyes and recited it from memory, in a singsong voice, "Judge not lest you be judged. Epilepsy, this Demon, is my home, and I am tired. I rest now. Hope and pray within yourself like Job. You will not stagger anymore. You will not fall anymore. You—"

"You refer to Job and the devil?" Bear interjected.

"Oh, yeah," she said, coming out of her reverie. "I have cassettes I've made on epilepsy and every book of the Bible." She feels called upon to educate the public about epilepsy. Bear agrees that Gloria, as one who actually has TLE, is the best person to describe and explain it, better surely than a doctor who has never had even one seizure. He also thinks that her grandiosity and messianic impulses are features of Geschwind's syndrome.

"Mrs. Johnson travels with her satchel full of cassettes of her reflections and meditations," he added, gesturing toward the stuffed handbag at her feet. In an article about personality and TLE, he wrote that Gloria initially presented him with "more than twenty spiral notebooks filled with somber personal reflections, religious exegeses and angry diatribes against former physicians, police and politicians. She filled one seventy-page notebook. . . . Her efforts were all the more remarkable because she suffered painful and deforming rheumatoid arthritis which forced her to write with hand supports."

Bear took a deep breath. He had one more question for her. "Now, Mrs. Johnson, are you a good person? Sensitive?"

Gloria thought for a moment. Calmly, she replied, "I'm like Job," the biblical figure who worked to accept great suffering as the will of a just God. "But, Dr. Bear," she continued, with sudden feeling, her sad eyes glistening, "why don't you let that man Hinckley out of jail?"

"There's a certain warmth here," Bear said to the class, grinning. "It's very easy to get to know her." As he told a colleague, she is "a remarkably caring and sensitive individual."

Bear is not the only physician who has noticed Gloria's appeal. She can be impossible to deal with, but she has a charming side. "Sometimes it appears that behind her impulsive and active behavior a frightened and obedient soul is hiding," wrote a psychiatrist who treated her in 1962 after a suicide attempt. She seemed "very sensitive and very suspicious, irritable and impulsive. From her sensitivity it comes that she 'puts up a front,' because she does not want to be bothered. Very suspicious, because 'very many people betrayed' her. *Irritable all the time.* But behind that very soft."

After Bear's lecture, a few students lingered to talk with Gloria. Bear introduced them; Gloria smiled and shook hands. The mood was warm. Bear thanked her for her contribution to the class. Gloria's companion, Sister Mary, pushed her wheelchair out of the building, alongside the grassy quadrangle, down a ramp, and into the chaos of the city street. Squinting in the sunlight, the two women waited on the sidewalk for one of the vans that the state provides to its handicapped citizens. Gloria enjoyed her lecturing, but she was tired and eager to get home.

At Gloria's apartment house, a three-decker on a hill a few miles away, Sister Mary and the driver rolled her out of the van. Gloria stood up and shouted for Joe, a soft-spoken hospital janitor whom she married when she was thirty-five. Although they have lived apart for years, he still comes by most afternoons to cook her dinner and do her chores. Moments after her shout, a short, solidly built man in his late fifties emerged without a word from the building, folded the wheelchair, and carried it up the walkway to the covered porch. Gloria followed him slowly, groaning, gripping the railing with a gnarled hand. She said good-bye to Sister Mary, who stood chatting with Joe on the porch. Alone, Gloria made her way through the battered front door, labored up the flight of stairs to her apartment, and wrestled with her key in the door. "I don't feel right," she said. "Nothing's right."

Inside, she headed straight for the bedroom and dropped onto her bed. Because light can exacerbate her seizures, this small, wood-paneled room—where she spends the bulk of her time—is always kept dark. Heavy brocade curtains cover the windows. On this day, the only light sources were a small lamp casting a faint yellowy glow and a color television set, which she had left on. Flat surfaces were loaded with books, cassette tapes of her religious meditations, and spiral-bound notebooks containing her thoughts and notes about her work. *The Focus of Democracy*, in two volumes, and *Words of Eternal Life* lay atop a stack of Bibles. Glass animals, plastic flowers, and other knick-knacks adorned the ridged wainscoting. Framed letters from Bear and Bishop Riley, her diplomas and licenses in hairdressing, and pictures of Jesus Christ with the Sacred Heart and the Virgin Mary decorated the walls. A retouched photo of Gloria herself, taken when she was a dancer, wearing a scarlet overcoat with fur collar and a pillbox hat with an ostrich feather, hung above her bed. Covering the top of her dresser were bottles containing nail polish, Tums, Keri bath lotion, rubbing alcohol, Riopan antacid, Vicks Formula 44D, AquaPhor skin cream, and numerous prescription medications, including the anticonvulsants Dilantin and Mysoline. A foot-high plaster statue of Jesus, arms extended in blessing, stood among the medicines.

Joe soon brought in Gloria's dinner of baked chicken, white rice, and green peas. She ate little, drinking tea and smoking cigarettes instead.

Meanwhile, in Bear's office at the Deaconess Hospital near the campus of Harvard Medical School, he was dictating a letter to Gloria, which she would later read aloud, frame, and add to the collection of tributes hanging on her wall. "Dear Mrs. Johnson," he wrote, "Let me take this opportunity to thank you for your wonderfully gallant participation teaching medical students, interns, and residents, and most of all myself. . . . Neither the doctors nor the students understand as well as you the anguish of patients with TLE."

Gloria is expert in that anguish. Unlike Charlie and Jill, who developed TLE as adults, when its effects were overlaid on existing life-styles and personalities, Gloria has had frequent TLE seizures for more than fifty years, from the start of her conscious life. Bear and many other doctors who have treated her find it difficult to say where Gloria ends and TLE begins, a common problem with TLE that is unusually pronounced in Gloria. No one can disentangle her underlying personality from the effects of her TLE. She is an ordinary person who, unlike Charlie and Jill, does not seem ordinary; if anything, her story is reminiscent of van Gogh's. Like the artist, she turned to alcohol to dull the effects of her seizures; she committed numerous acts of violence toward others and toward herself; she was hospitalized on psychiatric wards for months; and she has an exaggerated version of Geschwind's syndrome. There the similarity ends.

No one knows why the syndrome appears to advantage in one person and to disadvantage in someone else. The reason may have nothing to do with epilepsy, but may instead reflect the underlying personality that epilepsy changes. Geschwind once said, "Epilepsy may alter the personality, may open the door, but [it] can never tell us what lies behind it." The actual mechanism by which TLE affects behavior—why the emotional extremes appear in one person as violence and hypersexuality, in another as emotional restraint—is a mystery. Less mysterious are the physical underpinnings of specific seizure states, such as Gloria's dizziness and nausea, Jill's visual hallucinations, and Charlie's experiences of *jamais vu*. While we do not fully understand the physiology of personality, we know a great deal about the source of discrete mental states in the brain.

CHAPTER FOUR

Mental States

The human brain does not give up its secrets without a struggle. In life, it has the look and feel of soft white cheese. It is laced with blood vessels, so that when cut in surgery, it resembles clumpy yogurt with strawberry sauce. It pulses; you can see the heart beat in it. Otherwise the living brain reveals little. Though it is composed of billions of nerve cells containing molecular structures through which electricity moves, it appears to have no moving parts.

In death, the brain becomes accessible. During every autopsy, a pathologist slices the back of the head from ear to ear, and she pulls the scalp forward so that it meets and then covers the face. She saws, roughly along the hairline, through the skull encasing the brain, and she removes the bony crown, about one-half inch thick. Inside the skull is a protective membrane, a dense skin called the *dura mater,* Latin for "tough mother." The pathologist cuts through this membrane to expose the brain, floating in its briny fluid. Reaching underneath the brain, she severs the spinal cord and the stringy nerves, veins, and arteries that attach the brain to the body. She pulls the brain from the remainder of the skull and ties a piece of twine to its base. For several weeks, the brain is suspended upside down in a plastic bucket containing formaldehyde, an arrangement that enables it to maintain its shape. Formaldehyde fixes and preserves the brain, while slightly altering its appearance and consistency. Its color goes from white to yellowish gray. The organ solidifies, becoming more like Gouda cheese, less like Brie. Its clefts and bulges gradually become firmer, until its surface looks like the outside of a basket, and it gives only slightly when pressed. As a result of these changes, the brain in the bucket reveals features that the living brain concealed.

Lifted from the bucket, the human brain weighs between three and four pounds. It is roughly the size and shape of a cauliflower, a squeezed oval rather than a perfect sphere. Like the human body, the brain is symmetrical. It has left and right halves, called cerebral hemispheres, which are shaped and oriented like walnut halves. Though the hemispheres are attached to each other by a few cables, they are otherwise distinct, and their functions are both shared and discrete. By means of nerve fibers that cross near the center of the brain, each hemisphere controls the opposite side of the body. In most people, the left hemisphere operates serially, taking the lead in functions that rely on details, such as language, numerical calculations, and dexterity, while the right hemisphere operates holistically, leading in functions that rely on contour, such as emotion, visual perception, and spatial orientation. Researchers are able to demonstrate these functional divisions in a living person by injecting a barbiturate that temporarily depresses the activity of one hemisphere and asking the subject to perform various tasks. With the right hemisphere shut down, most people cannot move the left side of their body; they ignore the left side of space; they cannot copy simple line drawings; and they have difficulty reading facial expressions or behaving appropriately in company. With the left hemisphere depressed, most people are unable to move their right side, recall a list of numbers, speak, or read.

These functional divisions are not entirely built in. Early in life, the cerebral hemispheres are relatively flexible: either can develop to assume most of the functions of both, so that a child born with only one hemisphere can grow up to be relatively normal. As an adult, she may be weak or paralyzed on the side opposite the missing hemisphere, but her spatial awareness, emotions, and language are likely to be intact.

This functional plasticity does not last. If an adult loses one hemisphere, in surgery for epilepsy or tumor or as a result of a massive stroke, the remaining hemisphere can no longer assume the functions of the missing half. Huge deficits, both physical and mental, result. If the right hemisphere is lost or damaged, the person is unable to control the left side of his body, is unaware of the left side of space, and expresses emotions inappropriately. Yet his use of language is normal in the sense that he can read and understand speech. If the left hemisphere is lost or damaged, the person's emotions and sense of space remain normal, but the right side of his body is paralyzed and he is unable to speak, read, or comprehend language. In spite of these functional differences, the two hemispheres look alike.

Each hemisphere is divided into four sections called lobes. The four pairs of lobes—frontal, occipital, parietal, and temporal—are located, respectively, in the front, rear, top, and bottom of each hemisphere. Though rounded and protruding while growing from the bulb of the brain during fetal development, these lobes are in maturity almost continuous sections of each hemisphere's semisolid mass. The division of each hemisphere into lobes is not apparent in the living brain, and it is only subtly apparent at autopsy. Despite their fuzzy boundaries, the lobes serve as compass points to doctors, who refer to brain regions as, for instance, "occipitotemporal," meaning located where the occipital and temporal lobes adjoin.

While many functions require the cooperation of several lobes, some regions are devoted to particular tasks. Hughlings Jackson's idea that epileptic scars are located in regions controlling the function affected in seizures led to the theory of "localization of function," which posits that movement, sensation, memory, and language are specific to certain brain regions. Penfield and Jasper, in the course of operating on hundreds of patients with TLE, mapped the "strips" of brain tissue devoted to movement and sensation, which lie at the juncture of the frontal and parietal lobes. As a graphic representation of what they had found, the doctors drew for each set of functions a "homunculus," or little person, whose body parts were proportional to the amount of brain tissue devoted to the operation of each part. The motor homunculus had huge lips and hands, a tiny torso, and no genitals or nose. In contrast, the sensory homunculus had a huge tongue and hands, a sizable torso, genitals, and a nose. Other parts of the temporal, parietal, and frontal lobes control language; damage to or removal of these regions causes problems with language comprehension or speech. In fact, each pair of lobes is now associated with one or several specialized functions, which go haywire when that pair is damaged or removed.

Inside the forehead are the frontal lobes, extending back several inches to a fissure that runs nearly vertically inside a person's temples. The frontal lobes contain tissues devoted to speech, movement, and abstract thought. They are considered the administrators of the human brain because they control high-level analysis and sorting of the information that arrives from the world and from the other lobes as a confusion of sounds, images, sensations, and feelings. A person with frontal-lobe damage has trouble distinguishing the trivial from the important. If a doctor asks a patient to repeat the sentence, "It's snowing outside," and the patient replies, "I can't, because it's not," she probably has frontal-lobe damage. When the frontal lobes are severely damaged, as in a prefrontal leucotomy, or "lobotomy," the infamous twentieth-century surgical treatment for schizophrenia, a person loses all initiative and becomes unable to carry out the basic act of choosing to urinate in private, much less the complex act of designing a house.

In the back of the head, above and behind the scruff of the neck, are the occipital lobes. (*Occiput* is Latin for "back of the head.") The most specialized pair of lobes in the brain, these are devoted to vision.

Just beneath the crown of the head are the parietal lobes—*parietal* is Latin for "within walls." These lobes control sensation, spatial orientation, and certain features of language and memory.

At the base of the parietal lobes is a deep, nearly horizontal cleft. Below that, sitting atop the spinal column and roughly between the ears, are the regions controlling hearing and smell, learning and memory, and emotions and drives—the temporal lobes, whose name comes from the Latin *tempus*, or "the sides of the skull."

To see the entire temporal lobes, as with the other lobes, the pathologist must slice into the brain. The bulk of each lobe is hidden from view, folded and layered into a mass that extends from the surface several inches deep. Slices are made on planes parallel to the face. Each cross section includes portions of both temporal lobes and, depending on the location, of several other lobes. Each slice resembles a cross section of the trunk of a tree. It is more or less round, with a scalloped edge, a whitish center (the brain's "white matter"), and a darker rim about one-quarter inch thick. The rim is the "gray matter," also known as "cortex," which derives from the Latin word for "bark." Cerebral cortex, or gray matter, is essential to performing high-level functions such as thinking, speaking, and skillful movements. Perhaps the most complex tissue in existence, gray matter appears in greatest quantity in creatures highest in the evolutionary chain. Scarce in reptiles, it is more plentiful in humans than in lower mammals. Since gray matter exists only on the brain's surface, the surface of a human brain must be relatively larger than the surfaces of other animals' brains. Nature accomplishes this feat by folding and layering the human brain, to increase the area of its surface. In the cross section of the human temporal lobes, the cortex is tucked and pleated like a skirt.

So far, the temporal-lobe slice resembles slices of the other lobes. All four lobes have similar shapes. All are composed of white matter surrounded by gray. But the temporal lobes are different in an important respect. Near the center of the temporal-lobe slice is a region of darker, variegated shapes. Unique among the brain's lobes, the temporal lobes have this extra component, the limbic system, at their core.

The limbic system is a bunch of structures consisting of both gray and white matter that lies at a spot near the center of the brain. The name derives from the system's placement and shape: *limbus* is Latin for "border" or "fringe"; this system loops around the spinal cord and the corpus callosum, the fibrous cable connecting the cerebral hemispheres, to make a sort of *C* on a horizontal plane inside the temporal lobes. While doctors argue over its exact borders, most agree that the limbic system contains some of the oldest brain structures, including the amygdala, hippocampus, mammillary bodies, and anterior thalamus, and that it participates in such varied functions as memory, hormone production, the sleep-wake cycle, smell, and the determination of appropriate emotional response. It is your limbic system that decides whether you will run, flirt, or fight. When you come upon a rabbit on a wooded path and the rabbit runs, the animal's limbic system has worked. Gone awry, the limbic system can cause a creature to fight when others would run, or to attempt sexual intercourse when others would feel shame or hide. The limbic system is found in the brains of all animals. A crocodile brain is almost entirely limbic. The functional part of a human infant's brain is largely limbic. An adult human brain is only partly limbic, the balance being devoted to higher functions such as language and thought.

The limbic system and the temporal lobes work together and are sometimes called the temporolimbic region, which David Bear referred to in his Harvard Medical School lecture as "the emotional brain." Since temporal lobe epilepsy can result from impairment of both the temporal lobes and the limbic system, it is sometimes called temporolimbic epilepsy, which shrinks to the same acronym, TLE. Partial, or focal, seizures can occur practically anywhere in the brain, but they are most likely to start in the temporolimbic region. The reason may be that the tissue of this region, which is also involved in learning, is unusually lively and therefore more likely than other parts of the brain to seize.

Like the rest of the brain, the temporolimbic region is composed of vast numbers of cells. Among these are neurons, or nerve cells, a type of cell peculiar to the nervous system. The center of each neuron—its cell body—lies at the surface of the brain. Many cell bodies packed together compose the cortex, or gray matter, the outer rim of brain tissue. The pinkish-gray color of these cell bodies gives the gray matter its name.

Extending from each cell body is a long, whitish tentacle called an axon. Light in color because of their fatty coating, axons constitute the brain's "white" matter. They link neurons to each other, enabling them to communicate. By interconnecting billions of neurons in a complex communication network, axons send messages around the brain. Individual axons can be several feet long; like telephone cables, they join to make thick bundles, crisscrossing the brain.

The force that travels down axons, allowing neurons to communicate, is electricity. Electric current is produced by chemical changes occurring inside and outside neurons, in a process known as "firing." Once produced, the current travels from the cell body down its axon, jumps across the gap between it and a dendrite, or branch, of an adjacent neuron, then moves through that neuron. The chemical message carried by the current may be sufficient to cause the second neuron to fire or, if it was firing already, to cease its activity. In other words, the firing of one neuron can turn other neurons "on" or "off." Neurons whose messages customarily turn other neurons on are "excitatory"; those that turn others off are "inhibitory."

To envision this submicroscopic process on a human scale, imagine that neurons are people, crowded tightly, shoulder to shoulder, on a field. If one person starts shaking—or one neuron fires—the people around him will shake a little, too. This movement passes along the crowd until it dissipates. Some people—excitatory neurons—shout and flail when jostled. This intensifies the shaking and speeds its passage along. Other people—inhibitory neurons—are calm. When shaken, they hardly react, and the shaking subsides. The environment also affects the crowd's response. If the weather on the field is comfortable, excitable people may stay calm. But if the temperature is extremely hot or cold, even calm people may become jittery enough to pass along the shaking. The neural equivalents of extreme weather conditions on the field include the brain's overall chemical environment, the firing of adjacent networks, or a nearby seizure focus.

As Jackson suspected, the brain appears to consist of a series of these networks, or circuits, each with a particular role. Recognizing an object as a car, for instance, is thought to require several networks that take information from various parts of the brain: one part to convey the car's image, another part to compare that image to remembered shapes, and a third part to identify and name it. If an entire network of neurons is turned on, the electrical message moves through many neurons to many parts of the brain, turning successive neurons on and off. Such a chain of firing neurons is at the base of every ordinary action, feeling, or thought.

It is widely accepted that every human endeavor is the result of the activation of electrical circuits in the brain, but no one knows exactly how this process occurs. The workings of neuronal circuits are complex, and only their rough outlines are understood. We know that neurons in several lobes are required for even simple mental states. We know that neurons in one lobe are frequently a part of many neural networks. But we do not know the mechanism by which electrical activity becomes a thought.

We do know, however, what prompts neuronal firing. In ordinary experience, there are two prompters of the electrical impulse. The first is intention. When you will your arm to move, a network of neurons in your motor cortex fires, sending a command to your arm muscles, and your arm moves. In this way, you have mental control over much brain function: you can gesture, remember events and equations, and feel certain emotions at will.

The second ordinary prompter is events in the outside world. If, while you are driving, a traffic light turns from green to yellow, a neural network usually fires to make you stop the car. If a truck suddenly moves dangerously close to you, other neural networks fire, making you swerve away. This happens automatically, before you have a chance to formulate an intention or a thought.

But there is another prompter of neuronal firing that is rare in normal experience. This is a seizure, in which normal networks fire abnormally, without the ordinary internal or external causes. For no apparent reason, a person suddenly has an experience—a sense of panic, a jerk of her arm, or a childhood memory. During the seizure the mind is unaccountably split in two: one part realizes the experience is seizural; another part feels the experience is real. This is what happened to Charlie during his big seizure in the woods, when he existed simultaneously in the ordinary world and the world of dreams.

The cause of this dual awareness has been explored by Marcel Kinsbourne, a behavioral neurologist who studies the physical correlates of human behavior, or what happens in the nervous system during feelings, actions, and thoughts. A tall man with fine features and a British accent, Kinsbourne was born in Vienna in 1931, was educated at Oxford, spent a year practicing at the Queen Square hospital in London, and now works at the Eunice Kennedy Shriver Center outside Boston. One spring day,

seated in his office, which smells vaguely of pipe smoke and is
decorated with pictures of children at play, he explained the neural activity underlying dual awareness. "In a seizure," he said,
"the ordinary neural pattern stops, a second neural pattern
comes and goes away again, and then the first one resumes, and
you say, 'What just happened to me?'" The experience is like having a smaller brain inside the actual brain that now and then
takes over for a while, compromising the integrity of a person's
behavior and experience.

Kinsbourne contrasted this experience of a seizure to ordinary experience. "Normally," he said, "everything in the brain
occurs in a coordinated manner, with all the elements fitting in
place, interacting with each other. For instance, right now my
experience is unified. I am in my office, I am talking, I have
some thoughts in my mind, I am holding my pipe in one hand
and my matches in the other, and I have the intention of lighting
this pipe at some point. None of this is conflicting, because it's
all orderly, it has priorities, and nothing comes out of nowhere.
But imagine how a disorganized brain [during a seizure] might
separately view itself conversing and holding matches in one
hand, and then suddenly wonder, 'Why am I holding matches?'
The matches wouldn't be tied in to the conversation, so they
wouldn't seem to make sense." A TLE seizure provides the neural basis for the lack of coordination in that brain.

Despite its abnormal prompter, the seizure consists of
snatches of ordinary feelings, actions, or thoughts. "You can't do
something in a seizure that you couldn't otherwise do," Kinsbourne continued, returning his unlit pipe to his mouth. A
seizure is "a fragment of normal behavior that occurs out of context because the irritability of nerve cells causes them to fire too
often, outside the usual controls. Neurons can do one of two
things: they can fire either slower or faster than the normal
state." If neurons fire more slowly or stop, that creates a
"deficit," meaning the loss of a function. If neurons fire much
faster than the normal state, that creates a seizure. In a seizure,
Kinsbourne explained, "a behavior or behaviors are wrenched
away from their adaptive context because of disease—because
the patterns of neurons that generate the behavior are simply
overready to fire spontaneously."

These neurons fire spontaneously because they have "a

pathologically lowered threshold for discharging," or a "seizure threshold," the point at which any neuron will fire abnormally. Since everyone has neural networks and electrical activity in the brain, everyone has the equipment necessary for a seizure to occur. Marc Dichter, a neurologist, notes that the "ease and rapidity [with which seizures occur suggest that] the normal brain . . . contains within its . . . structure a mechanism which is inherently unstable and which can be influenced in many different ways to produce a seizure." Factors that can lower anyone's seizure threshold include electrical stimulation of the brain, hyperventilation, sleep deprivation, and ingestion of drugs, including alcohol, cocaine, and lysergic acid diethylamide (LSD). Alcohol withdrawal can cause seizures even in nonepileptics; these attacks, known as "rum fits," consist of hallucinations, delirium, and bodily convulsions, and occur days or weeks after a binge. Some TLE patients report that the mental effort of chanting or prayer can bring on seizures. In rare cases, patients have "reflex epilepsy," in which seizures are set off by repetitive sounds or images, such as ringing bells or flashing strobe lights. Whatever the reason, whenever the electrical activity in the brain exceeds its seizure threshold, a seizure begins. The difference between people with epilepsy and everyone else, then, is the relative height of their seizure thresholds: people with epilepsy are simply more likely than others to seize. The reason may be partly hereditary: in 1991, researchers working with mice found a gene responsible for temporolimbic seizures, and they predicted future identification of a human "epilepsy gene."

The cause of the lowered seizure threshold, as Jackson realized, is a scar that alters the electrical activity in part of the brain. Exactly how the scar creates discharge sufficient to exceed the threshold and start a seizure is not known. In most cases, the scar results from a physical or chemical insult to the brain, which can occur before birth, as in Jill, during birth, as in Gloria, or after birth, as in Charlie. The seizures that develop over the scar do not constitute a disease per se; rather, they are symptoms of the damaged brain. Moreover, seizures are not random. Although they bypass intention, they are learned. Once certain neural pathways fire abnormally, they are more likely to do so again. A network of such neurons is known as a seizure focus.

The location of the scar, Jackson also realized, determines the seizural effects. Doctors use their observations of these effects and their knowledge of brain function to pinpoint a patient's scar, where seizure activity starts. If located, the scar can sometimes be removed, as in Penfield's surgical patients in Montreal. But often it is not possible on the basis of the seizure state to determine the lobe or even the hemisphere containing the scar. This is because during TLE seizures the discharge often spreads to the opposite or a neighboring lobe by means of numerous intricate connections between the temporolimbic region and the rest of the brain. In many cases, doctors look to EEG results and "physical signs"—such as unusual skills and handedness, which indicate hemispheric strengths, and bodily asymmetries, which indicate hemispheric weaknesses—in their attempt to locate a patient's scar.

In Gloria's case, the picture of the brain damage underlying seizures is relatively clear. The powerful emotions, spatial disorientation, and left-body movements during her seizures indicate involvement of her right hemisphere, which controls emotions, spatial orientation, and the left side of the body. Her body signs and most of her EEGs provide further evidence that the brain damage she suffered at birth was in her right hemisphere. Her right-handedness suggests a healthy left hemisphere. Her EEGs, when abnormal, show a major seizure focus in her right frontotemporal region and minor abnormalities in her right temporolimbic region and her left temporal lobe, the latter resulting, Bear presumes, from the spread of epileptic activity from the right-hemisphere seizure focus. Such spreading into her left hemisphere, which controls discrete information, may cause her tendency to confuse numbers and names. The relative size of the ventricles, the cavities that hold the brain's fluid, in her temporal region also displays a right-brain abnormality: on a brain scan done when she was in her thirties, her right temporal ventricle appeared enlarged, indicating that her right temporal region had atrophied, probably because of the brain damage that occurred at her birth.

The nature and location of Jill's brain damage is less clear, perhaps because it occurred so early in the development of her brain. Her smells and powerful seizural emotions suggest the involvement of her limbic system. Her hallucinations of colors and lights indicate seizure activity near the occipital lobes, where vision is controlled, and their placement in her right visual field suggests left-hemisphere epileptic activity. Her attacks of *jamais vu*, dreamy states, and Alice-in-Wonderland symptoms—the "fading out" and "floating" feelings—come from upper temporal regions near the parietal lobes; because they involve her sense of space, they probably involve the right hemisphere. So her seizures point to diffuse epileptic activity in her temporolimbic, occipitotemporal, and temporoparietal regions, possibly in both hemispheres. Her EEGs show evidence of abnormalities in both hemispheres, more often in the left than in the right. Schomer suspects that in her, as in Gloria, seizure discharge may spread from one temporolimbic region to the other. The hemisphere where seizures start is likely to be the one that was damaged by DES before her birth, although both hemispheres may have been damaged, or the focus in one may have spawned a second focus in the other, as sometimes happens with TLE. Her strong right-hemisphere skills—her tremendous intuition about people and situations—indicate an unusually dominant right hemisphere, suggesting that DES damaged her left hemisphere. Her difficulties remembering numbers and words since developing TLE also point to damage in her left hemisphere, which controls numerical calculations and verbal memory. If her left hemisphere was damaged in the womb, this could explain her remarkable right-hemisphere strengths, because early damage to one hemisphere often causes the other to overcompensate, so that unusual skills are one possible result of brain injury. Her physical signs—right-handedness, an asymmetric smile caused by a smaller left side of the face, and a slight weakness of the left hand—confuse the picture by indicating a dominant left hemisphere, which contradicts her cognitive strengths and most of her EEGs. Schomer suspects that epileptic activity from the initial damage in her left hemisphere spread over the years into her healthier right hemisphere. In the uncertainty over her brain damage Jill is not alone among Schomer's TLE patients, in a third of whom he cannot determine even the hemisphere where seizures start.

Charlie, with the least severe TLE, has the most questions about the location of his scar. His seizural effects indicate involvement of temporal, parietal, and occipital lobes. His dreamy states and memory problems come from temporal regions controlling memory and consciousness. His "funny feelings"—bodily malaise and stomach and head pains—indicate involvement of parietal regions. His flashing lights are occipito-temporal. As to which hemisphere is affected first, his consistent right-handedness suggests a healthy left hemisphere, indicating that the suspected damage from his childhood encephalitis is in his right hemisphere. The slight shrinkage of features on the left side of his face and the unusually brisk reflexes that Waddington found on the left side of his body also suggest right-hemisphere damage. Further evidence that the scar is right-sided is that the function most often affected during his seizures, spatial orientation, is controlled by the right hemisphere, while his speech, a left-hemisphere function, is never affected. Yet the results of his EEGs are inconsistent: some show problems in the right hemisphere, while others indicate abnormalities mainly in the left. All show diffuse abnormalities, both temporolimbic and temporofrontal. Edwards thinks that during seizures Charlie's epileptic activity spreads rapidly from wherever it begins into the opposite hemisphere.

Since seizures are composed of ordinary mental states, they can take almost any form. According to Paul Spiers, TLE seizures "cover all the categories of human existence and processing of the environment." To lend order to the multiplicity of seizure symptoms, Spiers has divided them into six categories, which he identifies as hallucinatory, emotional, autonomic (referring to bodily functions outside conscious control), motor, sensory, and experiential. Hallucinatory seizure symptoms consist of tastes, smells, sounds, voices, and visions of colors, lights, or menacing figures. Emotional symptoms span the spectrum of human emotional states, including attacks of panic or anger, explosions of tears or laughter, and orgasm. Physical states such as irregular heartbeat, shortness of breath, dizziness, flushing, and vomiting are among the autonomic symptoms. Lip smacking, undressing in public, staring, twitching, and transient paralysis are some of the motor seizure symptoms, as are "Jacksonian seizures" (named in honor of Jackson by Freud's teacher Charcot), which consist of tremors spreading up or down one side of the body. Sensory seizure symptoms include pain; the temporary inability to feel pain; and "paresthesias," bizarre feelings that patients report during seizures, such as "pins and needles," "bugs crawling" under the skin (formication), the sensation that a limb has been lost, the "Alice in Wonderland" symptoms in which objects seem to contract or expand (metamorphopsia) or the person seems to be falling down a hole, and even memories of sensations, such as of an arm being submerged in icy water. The final category, experiential symptoms, covers such alterations of consciousness as dreamy states; flashbacks; trances; automatisms; *déjà* and *jamais vu*; the sense that time is standing still or rushing by; the illusion of a presence, a döppelganger, or a "double" (such as Dostoevsky described in his short novel *The Double*); the feeling of being possessed; and mind-body dissociation, or depersonalization, in which the mind seems to separate from the body.

While TLE seizures are as varied as human behavior, the seizures of any individual tend to remain the same, time after time. "Across the population at large, seizures tap the whole wealth of human memory and experience," Kinsbourne said, "but *within the individual*, seizures are very idiosyncratic. When somebody has a seizure with temporal-lobe coloring, there's a limited repertoire of things that keep coming up in that individual. He may hear a certain song or church bells ringing; the next time he has a seizure, he's not hearing bongo drums, he's still hearing those stupid church bells." The seizure state "is very limited and crude and primitive. It's like a cognitive jerk. It's a little routine that runs off—a feeling, a smell, or an image. The seizure is always simpler, more limited, more rigid" than ordinary experience.

Van Gogh's typical seizure apparently involved stomach distress, panicky anger, a complex automatism—such as stalking Gauguin or disrobing in public—and perhaps, as the celestial pinwheels in *The Starry Night*, painted at Saint-Rémy the year before he died, might suggest, hallucinatory flashes of light.

Jackson's wife, Elizabeth, usually had a dreamy state, as does Charlie. Dostoevsky felt ecstasy and psychic pain. Gloria smells "burnt feces," or something equally unpleasant, and has automatisms. Penfield's patient Sylvère felt himself rotating and heard a voice calling his name. Jill has sensory hallucinations and feels a dread that she can neither rationalize nor stop. The reason for an individual's limited seizural repertoire is thought to be the way in which epileptic discharge moves through the brain. Abnormal firing is thought to follow the same few neural pathways in an individual each time a seizure occurs. Many TLE seizures involve multiple brain functions, including those not controlled by the temporal lobe, because the path of the firing often crosses several parts of the brain.

In the mind of the patient, the experience of a seizure is often no different from the same experience occurring normally. When Charlie feels lost during a seizure, for instance, his confusion is genuine; despite his familiarity with the area, he cannot find his way home. When Jill has a panic attack, the panic feels real. The only difference between it and normal panic, as when she was mugged, is contextual: in the seizure, there is no mugger present to prompt her fear. Similarly, the experience of an orgasm in a seizure and an ordinary orgasm is practically the same, according to twelve women with TLE studied in Canada in 1981. The only difference is that the seizural orgasms are unannounced and unwilled, lacking the normal period of arousal. Otherwise, the twelve patients in the study used ordinary terms to describe their seizural orgasms. A secretary said that during seizures she had a "fine feeling" that was "identical" to how she felt while masturbating, after which she felt terror and saw visions of "two-headed beasts, elephants, rhinoceroses, and hippopotamuses, running around in circles but making no noise." (These seizures ceased after a right temporal lobectomy.) Another woman's seizural orgasms occurred in clusters during the days prior to menstruation. She felt discomfort and "a sensation of increasing warmth." Her mind blurred and her body went limp. She had an orgasm and then "a great sensation of calm," during which she had "increased vaginal secretions." A third patient, a nurse's aide, said her orgiastic seizures were premenstrual and nocturnal.

She felt sexually aroused, breathed deeply and fast, and briefly lost consciousness; then, she said, "I come in my pants." A male patient not included in the study reported having a seizural orgasm whenever he saw a safety pin. Over time, he told his doctors, he learned to bring on such a seizure simply by imagining a pin.

Among the experts, however, there is controversy over the difference between a normal state and the same state occurring abnormally, in a seizure. Schomer, a specialist in electroencephalography who reads the EEG during temporal lobectomies at Boston's Beth Israel Hospital, is one of the doctors who believe the distinction is clear. Born in Chicago in 1946 and trained at the Montreal Neurological Institute, Schomer has the pale, round face of a baker in a children's tale, brown hair cut in a bowl shape, and a mild, avuncular air. Not long ago, seated behind the desk in his spotless office overlooking the Charles River, he stated that there is a visible difference between the EEGs of a seizure state and of the equivalent normal state.

If electrodes could be placed deep enough in the brain of a person during a seizure, Schomer said, the EEG would always look different from a nonepileptic's EEG. Seizure activity characteristically appears as a series of jagged spikes, which electroencephalographers call hypersynchronous discharge because the neurons are discharging in a more synchronous manner than they do during a normal state. "As part of her seizure, one of my patients does this," Schomer said, twisting his torso and arms to his right as if raising an invisible banner. When she does so, seizure activity appears on her EEG. If she made the same movement intentionally, however, seizure activity would not appear. Neither seizure activity, which is intermittent, nor the underlying spike focus—the continuous pattern that indicates abnormal electrical activity over the spot where seizures start— is within a person's control. What makes a seizure a seizure is its abnormal trigger, that mysterious third prompter of neuronal firing. Anyone can mimic a seizure state, but no one, including TLE patients themselves, can mimic the brain activity underlying it. No one can will an abnormal EEG.

Generalizing from this, Schomer attributed the difference between normal events and seizural ones to the degree of personal control. To remember a moment from your childhood is usually an act of will; to remember it during a seizure is unwilled. During the time that the brain disorder compromises the will, the brain—not the individual—is temporarily in control. As Gustave Flaubert wrote in 1857, thirteen years after he was diagnosed with TLE, his seizures arrived as "a whirlpool of ideas and images in my poor brain, during which it seemed that my consciousness, that my *me* sank like a vessel in a storm." Schomer explained that during a seizure "the individual does not have major influence" over what happens in his brain. While ordinary people "can control what brain pathways are used at any point in time, during seizures epileptics cannot." As a consequence, the actions that epileptics take during seizures are usually sudden, unplanned, and undirected, like van Gogh's clumsy self-mutilations and Gloria's unprovoked outbursts. Edwards remarked, "If the seizural behavior is violent, it's random throwing of things and flailing, rather than the purposeful act of robbing a bank or putting a knife to somebody's back so as to steal his wallet. During a seizure, a person may shout, spit, or scratch, but he is unlikely to rob a bank or break into a car. People who rape grandmothers and steal hubcaps are generally not neurological patients, because that's purposeful behavior."

Despite Schomer's stated certainty about the difference between TLE states and normal states, the limitations of the EEG prevent him from pinpointing any physical evidence of it. The damage that leads to TLE is usually too far within the brain to be accessible to the ordinary EEG. The commonly used electrode—called a surface electrode because it is placed on the scalp—receives information mainly from outer brain areas. Searching for a seizure focus in the temporolimbic region with surface electrodes is a little like listening through a wall to a conversation on the far side of the next room.

Most hospitals still rely on the ordinary EEG when TLE is suspected, but a few, such as Schomer's hospital, use special "depth electrodes," placed inside the brain by a surgeon. Nevertheless, depth electrodes often show no abnormalities in the temporal lobes, even when the person is seizing. EEGs give only a gross sense of what is going on in the brain, displaying the overall activity of hundreds of thousands of neurons rather than pinpointing the relatively few cells in which seizure activity may occur. The first EEG often shows no abnormalities: in patients with likely epilepsy of any kind, the first EEG is abnormal 29–50 percent of the time, and subsequent EEGs show abnormalities 59–92 percent of the time. Doctors agree that no test is an absolute indicator of the presence or absence of TLE: a positive EEG usually indicates epilepsy, but a negative EEG does not rule it out. In fact, many patients with strong diagnoses of TLE based on their recurrent seizure states and their fine response to anticonvulsant drugs do not have a positive EEG; roughly one-third of Schomer's TLE patients fall into this category.

While some experts like Schomer are confident in their assumption that there is a distinction between seizural and normal states, others are not so sure. One is Jill's therapist and Schomer's colleague, the neuropsychologist Spiers. In 1987, while lecturing on TLE to graduate and medical students in Boston, Spiers pointed out that most ordinary people have seizural experiences and that occasional paranormal states common in seizures, such as out-of-body experiences, distortions of space and time, and incorporeal voices, are common as well in the population at large. If not actual seizures, these experiences, according to Spiers, reflect abnormal electrical activity in the same regions as in TLE. "How many of you in this room," he asked his audience, "have had a *déjà vu*?" More than half of the forty people in attendance raised their hands. "Welcome, fellow epileptics," chuckled Spiers, a thirty-six-year-old Montreal native with a confident manner and swept-back blond hair. *Déjà vu* is common in the general population. Similarly, many nonepileptics report feelings of a presence. "You walk into your house," Spiers said, "and you're standing in a room with the TV on, and all of a sudden you get this funny feeling that someone's watching you." He scanned the room expectantly and added, "Many of us have had that experience. That's just what a seizure is like, only the seizure is more intense and prolonged." Another seizure state Spiers himself has is a high-pitched sound in his ear. "Now, we all have these experiences," he said. "Does that mean we all have seizures?" Several in his audience shook their heads. "Probably, it does," Spiers corrected. "We probably *all* have seizures, but that does *not* mean that we all have a seizure disorder." Epilepsies, or seizure disorders, consist of seizures that recur, not simply the incidental one or two. Many people have occasional seizure states, but only people with epilepsy have these experiences regularly, every week or day.

No matter how rarely they occur, seizure states require explanation. An ordinary person who now and then experiences visions of figures, flashes of colors, or incorporeal voices might explain them by saying, "I saw an alien," "I visited another world," or "God spoke to me." Similarly, Jill could interpret the beautiful lights and colors she sees in seizures as signs of otherworldly beings, and Gloria could believe in the reality of the knocking sounds she hears in seizures and the voice saying, "You must die." In fact, a minority of patients refuse to take the anticonvulsant medications their doctors prescribe because the drugs deprive them of mystical or paranormal experiences that they enjoy. Most patients, however, are like Jill; if given the choice, she would keep her wonderful hallucinatory seizures but would gladly give up all her seizures in order to avoid the dread panic attacks.

A bestselling author living in Manhattan described recurrent out-of-body experiences that his doctor considered consistent with TLE. In 1986, Donald Klein, a professor of psychiatry at Columbia University and director of research at the New York State Psychiatric Institute, examined Whitley Strieber, listened to his accounts of periods of altered consciousness over several months, and told him that he might have TLE. Any one of Strieber's experiences—which involved vivid smells; visual and auditory hallucinations; intense emotions; rapid heartbeats; *jamais vu*; formiculation; the sensations of rising, falling, and turning; depersonalization; and partial amnesia—illuminates the functions in and around the temporolimbic region.

On the night after Christmas in 1985, Strieber, his wife, Anne, and their ten-year-old son were asleep in their isolated log cabin in the woods of central New York, where the family was spending the holiday. At some point during the night, as Strieber recalled later under hypnosis, he awoke with a start. Anne slept undisturbed at his side, but he felt sure that something was wrong.

He heard a strange sound, a "whooshing" and "swirling," as if a crowd of people were rushing around in the room below.

"The noise just didn't make sense." Strieber sat up in bed and then, oddly, lay back down, all the while feeling that his actions were out of his control. The door to his bedroom appeared to move. He sat up again, feeling "very uneasy. My heart started beating harder. . . . What could be moving the door?" Just then, a figure about 3½ feet tall emerged from behind the door. It wore a wide-rimmed hat and a suit of armor from neck to knees. Moments later, as the figure "came rushing into the room," Strieber could make out "two dark holes for eyes and a black down-turning line of a mouth." He became immobilized and experienced "blackness" for "an unknown period of time."

Then the figure seemed to multiply, and Strieber had an extended out-of-body experience, during which he felt he was being physically removed from his bedroom by a group of aliens who had total control over him. He panicked each time he was moved. "My fear would rise when they touched me. Their hands were soft, even soothing, but there were so many of them that it felt a little as if I were being passed along by rows of insects." Among the places the aliens took him was a "depression in the woods" where he found himself sitting, naked and cold. To his left sat a small creature wearing a "gray-tan body suit," and to his right was a blue-robed creature, "invisible except for an occasional flash of movement."

All of a sudden, Strieber felt himself being transported upward to a place in the sky from which he could see the woods "corkscrewing slowly to the right." He found himself seated on a bench in a small, domed chamber, where several creatures cradled him while others rapidly circled the room. He was "entirely given over to extreme dread. The fear was so powerful that it seemed to make my personality completely evaporate." He felt "absolutely helpless in the hands of these strange creatures." At the same time, he sensed "something quite beautiful . . . but I can remember little about it." His vision blurred, and his surroundings seemed unpleasantly unfamiliar, as in a *jamais vu*. "I was in a mental state that separated me from myself . . . I was reduced to raw biological response. It was as if my forebrain had been separated from the rest of my system, and all that remained was a primitive creature, in effect an ape. . . . My mind had become a prison."

One of the alien figures produced a small box containing a

needle that "glittered when I saw it out of the corner of my eye." Strieber became "crazed with terror. I argued with them. 'This place is filthy,' I remember saying." A great sadness overcame him, and he began to scream.

A creature with an "electronic" voice asked how she could help him stop screaming, and he surprised himself by responding, "You could let me smell you." At this suggestion, he felt ashamed. But another creature seemed to comply, extending his hand for Strieber to smell. Its odor, which "remained the most convincing aspect of the whole memory" because it seemed so "real," was like cardboard with an "organic sourness" and a cinnamon "overtone."

A "bang and a flash" occurred, during which the creatures performed an operation on his head. He felt like weeping and sank "into a cradle of tiny arms." He felt himself falling and tried to stop. Then he was lifted into another room, "or perhaps I simply saw my present surroundings differently." He was on an operating table in a small theater surrounded by a group of creatures on benches, watching him. Two figures drew his legs apart and inserted into his rectum a scaly, triangular mechanical device more than a foot long. "It seemed to swarm into me as if it had a life of its own." He felt he was being raped. "For the first time I felt anger." The device was withdrawn, and a creature made an incision in Strieber's right hand, causing no pain.

The next morning, Strieber awoke to "a distinct sense of unease." For weeks, he was irritable and depressed. His wife noticed "a dramatic personality change" in him. He became demanding and accusatory, traits he had never before displayed. Several months later he had an EEG with "nasopharyngeal" electrodes, placed at the back of the nose, which are "not very effective at detecting EEG abnormalities," according to Howard Blume, a neurosurgeon. This single test showed no abnormalities. During the recording, Strieber experienced no symptoms, which further reduced the possibility of finding signs of a disorder. An EEG with ordinary electrodes that Strieber had a year later was also normal, as was a CAT scan. However, an MRI (magnetic resonance imaging) brain scan showed "occasional punctate foci of high signal intensity" in his left temporoparietal region, suggesting scarring that could lead to TLE.

When Klein informed him that the next step in a diagnostic

workup for TLE was to spend several weeks in a hospital undergoing a long-term EEG with implanted depth electrodes, which increase the chance of finding temporolimbic discharge, Strieber demurred. By then he had read a good deal about TLE, including the novels of Dostoevsky, and decided that he could live with his symptoms. TLE, if he had it, had not severely disrupted his life. He could adjust to occasional memory lapses and periods of altered consciousness; perhaps he could even incorporate his new experiences into his work.

Already a successful fiction writer specializing in horror novels, including *Catmagic*, *The Hunger*, and *The Wolfen*, Strieber turned to composing what he termed a nonfiction account of visits from and abductions by extraterrestrial beings. The resulting book, *Communion: A True Story* (1987), for which a publisher paid a one-million-dollar advance, became a best-seller, and a feature film was made from it. Although some critics dismissed Strieber's "nonfiction" as invented, his alien creatures would be true in a medical sense if indeed they resulted from seizures: they would be the psychic representations of abnormal electrical activity in his brain.

Spiers and other TLE experts suspect that the contemporary fascination with mysticism and the paranormal—such as UFOs, alien sightings, out-of-body travel, ESP, past-life regressions, and reincarnation—may be the result of mild, undiagnosed TLE in the general population. After Strieber's first book came out, more than two thousand grateful readers wrote to him describing experiences much like his, which prompted a second book on aliens, *Transformation* (1988). Sitting in his spacious Greenwich Village apartment during a break from a book publicity tour, Strieber, an affable, middle-aged Texas native, said, "I get fifty letters some days, and they're all describing the same thing [that I experienced]. This thing is very widespread. Three-fourths of my readers are absolutely convinced that it's visitors or UFOs. Well, UFOs are what this culture thinks of, because of TV and all, but it's definitely *not* UFOs. And I see no evidence that the visitors are real physical beings. I haven't the faintest idea what they really are. What interests me is what I do with my perceptions, not their origin." In fact, "I resist explaining what happened to me." Nevertheless, he added, "It's a terribly important and fundamentally human experience—perceptions that come from the level of mind that isn't interrupted by the rational structures that animate most of our thought. It's a kind of memory, a form of perception, or a mechanism of consciousness, something inexplicable that the mind attaches an explanation to, probably the same thing that caused people to believe in the old gods and myths, in angels, resurrection, and even UFOs today." He concluded, "It probably starts in the human mind."

A contemporary of Strieber's from Boston had similar experiences, which she interpreted as evidence of her possession by the devil until she was diagnosed with TLE. Over a twenty-year period, Mary Garth, a concert violinist and mother of three married to a college professor, regularly had extended automatisms with complex visual hallucinations, sexual sensations, and the feeling of being disconnected from herself. Unaware that these states could be seizures, she dealt with them by braiding them into narratives, which she recorded in her journal.

"I feel somewhat robotic, physically and emotionally insensitive, immune to stress, since I am not a part of life," she wrote of one seizure. "In a strange way, I feel immortalized. I am part of another dimension which cannot be described because it has no definition." In other seizures she sensed an evil presence and became extremely angry. She grabbed objects around her and threw them at people or walls, destroying her own and several friends' living rooms. If she was alone, she slashed her arms, legs, and back with razors, knives, and broken glass, never feeling any pain. Several times these feelings prompted her to dress up as a prostitute and prowl the streets of Boston in search of the "ugliest, dirtiest person" she could find with whom to have intercourse. On one occasion on the Fenway, a grassy swath of Boston frequented by joggers and drug pushers, police found her having intercourse with a derelict; she had told him to hold a knife to her throat and have sex with her. "I am led by some morbid, seductive force into my backyard," she wrote of the seizural feelings that inspired this kind of behavior. "The night is black. The moon is strangely charismatic. The trees are grim silhouettes against a gray horizon. The breeze kisses my naked body. I feel that I am having a sexual encounter with Satan. I experience a compelling and hypnotic fascination with Evil—but there is no pain." The loss of pain sensation during her seizures may have been the same symptom that enabled van Gogh to cut off part of his ear.

Mary's seizures began in her late teens, but they were not diagnosed until she was nearly forty. In the interim she, like countless other people with TLE, was misdiagnosed as psychotic. "At most hospitals today," Spiers explained, "if you show up in the emergency room complaining that you feel panic, you saw a vision of the Virgin Mary dripping blood, and you smelled a dead mouse"—all seizure symptoms—"you're not going to get diagnosed as epileptic. You're going to be called schizophrenic, and you're going to be sent straight to psychiatry." Schizophrenia, a common psychiatric disorder affecting roughly one in a hundred people, or two to three million Americans, is about as prevalent as the combined forms of epilepsy. It involves delusions, hallucinations, bizarre or incoherent behavior and thoughts, indifference, apathy, and withdrawal. "Some of the crazy behavior related to schizophrenia may be epileptic," according to Spiers. In the 1950s, he recalled, surgeons implanted depth electrodes in the brains of schizophrenics and discovered that "schizophrenics had spikes and discharges in their limbic systems when they were being crazy." While there is no cure for schizophrenia, drugs reduce some of its symptoms, supportive psychotherapy may help, and some schizophrenics eventually improve for unknown reasons.

Schizophrenia has no undisputed diagnostic marker, equivalent to the abnormal EEG during a seizure that clearly indicates TLE. Once thought to be solely the result of upbringing, schizophrenia is now believed to have biological, viral, and genetic causes as well. Brain scans show anatomic abnormalities in the temporal lobes of many schizophrenics, and at autopsy one in three schizophrenics' brains display further abnormalities, usually in the temporolimbic region. People whose mothers were exposed to the flu during the fifth month of pregnancy have an increased incidence of schizophrenia. Furthermore, the disease occurs more frequently in blood relatives of schizophrenics than in the general population.

TLE is often misdiagnosed not only as schizophrenia but also as mood disorders, according to John Kuehnle, a psychiatrist, who noted that TLE's widespread misdiagnosis "has unbelievable implications for psychiatry." Kuehnle estimated that 5 percent of people with affective disorders such as depression, manic-depressive illness, and mania "actually have TLE." He recalled one patient with the diagnosis of manic-depressive illness who did not improve when she was prescribed lithium, the usual treatment. Noting her religiosity—"she talked to Jesus every day and wrote religious treatises"—her regular blackouts, and her attacks of *déjà vu*, Kuehnle sent her for an EEG, which showed an epileptic focus in her right temporal lobe. When he prescribed a combination of electroconvulsive therapy, which is occasionally effective in treating TLE, and the anticonvulsant Tegretol, her condition improved. "Unless you ask the right questions of patients with TLE," he explained, "they may look like manic depressives, many of whom are hyperreligious." Similarly, he added, "fifteen to twenty percent of so-called schizophrenics, including many of the 'chronic residual schizophrenics' on the back wards of state hospitals who don't respond to traditional treatments for psychoses, are actually temporal lobe epileptics." According to Spiers, one-fourth to one-third of the TLE patients seen at Beth Israel Hospital during the 1980s had originally been diagnosed as having non-epileptic psychiatric disease.

During the years prior to Mary Garth's correct diagnosis, she spent many months in psychiatric hospitals, often in solitary confinement and on antidepressant or antipsychotic drugs, and she underwent regular electroconvulsive therapy, or ECT, popularly known as "shock treatments." Then when she was in her mid-thirties and a psychiatric inpatient at Massachusetts General Hospital, a doctor suspected TLE and called in Spiers and his Beth Israel colleagues as consultants on her case. While Spiers was doing a psychological test on her, she had a seizure. "All of a sudden she got this real evil look in her eye," he recalled. "She threw the cards used for the test in my face. She ran across the room, picked up her handbag, and threw that at me, too." Spiers yelled for help, nurses arrived to subdue her, and Mary seemed to calm down. Spiers and the nurses went out to the nursing station "to talk about how this was a perfect example of the seizures she has." Meanwhile, Mary was sneaking down the corridor in an attempt to leave the hospital and "find someone to have relations with." Spiers noted that when her condition was treated for the first time with the anticonvulsant medications Tegretol and Dilantin, she responded unusually well: her seizures ended and she was able to return to her musical career.

TLE seizures are difficult to recognize not only when they are so extreme as to seem psychotic, as in Mary, but also when they are covert or subtle or they mimic normal behavior. TLE can be a "hidden disease," Gloria explained. "You can see my arthritis— my hand is deformed, and I have trouble walking—but you can't see my TLE. You can't tell when I'm going to have a seizure, or if I do. I could be out socializing, and all of a sudden, boom, I seize. If I didn't tell people I was epileptic, they wouldn't know."

Further confusing the picture of diagnosis, according to Kinsbourne, is the fact that seizurelike states are prevalent in people who do not have epilepsy. In contrast to Schomer, who thinks that the loss of personal control is unique to epileptics during seizures, Kinsbourne believes that all people frequently act and feel without volition. "We are constantly seeing and hearing things that are not happening at all, because we expect them to," Kinsbourne said one day. Calling these experiences "unwilled cognitions," Kinsbourne smiled and said he had had an unwilled thought that very morning. "I woke up and I smelled tobacco, somebody smoking." But when he rose and looked around, no one was there. Then he realized the reason for his smell. "Now, today is Tuesday, but on Sunday mornings my gardener comes—early, quietly—and he smokes a cigarette. I know he is there because I can smell his cigarette smoke coming up into my bedroom, where I am still sleeping. This morning, I slept late, and for a moment it was *as if* it were Sunday. In that context, I could swear I smelled tobacco. I absolutely smelled it! Now, if the gardener had been accused of a crime, and I had to give testimony—Was he there?—I would say he *must* have been, because I smelled his tobacco! There was a momentary context which made this a highly probable experience. I didn't merely *think* I had this experience; I *had* it. I know it was baseless; it was like a hallucination; it comes under the category of hallucinations in sane people. But that makes it no less real than experiences which have a physical basis," such as seizures. "Memory does this all the time," he concluded, "and this is why eyewitness testimony is worthless."

The neurologist's experience calls to mind the moment in

Marcel Proust's *Remembrance of Things Past* when the adult narrator is jolted by a vivid childhood memory upon tasting a petite
madeleine dipped in tea. The narrator, named Marcel, is thought
to be based on Proust, whom the neurologist William Gordon
Lennox suspected of having undiagnosed TLE because of passages in his masterpiece. "I raised to my lips a spoonful of the
tea in which I had soaked a morsel of the cake," Marcel reports.
"No sooner had the warm liquid mixed with the crumbs touched
my palate than a shudder ran through me and I stopped, intent
upon the extraordinary thing that was happening to me. An
exquisite pleasure had invaded my senses, something isolated,
detached, with no suggestion of its origin. And at once the vicis-
situdes of life had become indifferent to me, its disasters innocuous, its brevity illusory—this new sensation having had on me
the effect which love has of filling me with a precious essence . . .
[and an] all-powerful joy. . . . And . . . in that moment all the
flowers in our garden . . . and the good folk of the village and
their little dwellings and the parish church and the whole of
Combray and its surroundings, taking shape and solidity, sprang
into being, town and gardens alike, from my cup of tea." This
resembles van Gogh's experience, described in a letter to his
brother, of his childhood home suddenly coming into his mind
in detail, down to a bird's nest in a nearby tree.

   Marcel's memory bursts upon him mysteriously, out of context and unwilled—like a seizure, except that its prompter is the
taste of the cake rather than abnormal electrical activity. Certain
neurons in Proust's narrator associate a taste with the village of
Combray, just as certain neurons in Kinsbourne associated
sleeping late with the smoke of the gardener's Sunday-morning
cigarette. Kinsbourne compared his own and Proust's "unwilled
cognitions" to the seizures that Penfield stimulated in surgical
patients on the operating table. "If someone puts an electrode on
your occipital lobe, you see flashing lights and whirling circles,
which you would normally see only if input were being transmit-
ted from the world through the eye. In both the unwilled cogni-
tion and the seizure, neurons discharge without being released
to do so by the usual means. But these unwilled cognitions happen absolutely all the time, based on expectancy. What's unusual
is when the experience produced by the discharge isn't
expected," as in a seizure.

Religious states also rely on expectancy but may resemble seizures, Kinsbourne said. "An apparition of the Virgin may be generated by one's intense expectancy and wish. When you expect something, you visualize it; your brain produces the image of what it would be like if it happened. There is a *patterned discharge* if I am expecting the Virgin Mary to come, and it's time, at any moment"—he narrowed his eyes and waved his hands as if perceiving the Virgin's approach—"and I can see her already before she comes." He explained, "An expectancy may be so great that if it's also fairly dark and murky, I can *see* that shape approaching. If somebody wants it that much, he may experience it. The intense expectancy releases the experience."

The closer one approaches the dividing line between normal and abnormal states, the more the terrain shifts. "Normal" and "abnormal" begin to seem no more than labels for things that no one understands. "The interesting question," Kinsbourne observed, "is, What else can generate patterned brain activity other than the input that is supposed to, or the expectancy that often does? I don't have an answer to that. With TLE, sometimes the pathological discharge can be quite complex; it can release very highly patterned activity over a short period of time; *something* is triggering that. Whether it's the same thing that triggers that in you and me when we occasionally have a *déjà vu*, I don't know. I have great difficulty defining where this sort of thing stops, and the seizure starts."

Numerous reported seizures incorporate religious states. Spiers tells of a woman with TLE whose seizures consist of a hallucination in her right visual field of a statue of the Virgin Mary, "its fingers cut off, dripping blood, telling her to harm herself." The author and broadcaster Karen Armstrong, a former nun who has "apprehended" God in TLE seizures, described the experience: "Suddenly everything comes together in a moment—everything adds up, and you're flooded with a sense of joy, and you're just about to grasp it, and then you lose it and you crawl into an attack. . . . It's easy to see how, in a prescientific age, an epileptic or any temporal lobe fringe experience like that could be thought to be God Himself."

Joan of Arc, the French farm girl who became a saint, from age thirteen reported ecstatic moments in which she saw flashes of light, heard voices—of Saints Margaret, Michael, and Catherine—and saw visions of angels. In the opinion of the neurologist Lydia Bayne, these states were "seizures—experiences of ineffable bliss in which she felt that the secrets of the universe were about to be revealed to her," and they were set off by the ringing of church bells. Joan's voices and visions propelled her to become a soldier in the effort to save France from English domination and led to her martyrdom in 1431, when she was nineteen.

Other mystical states may have neurological causes. "It is usually difficult," the physician Macdonald Critchley wrote, "to distinguish between actual visions and less tangible mental and spiritual impressions of a presence." To illustrate this difficulty, Critchley mentioned the phenomena detailed by Saint Teresa of Jesus, which are consistent with hallucinatory TLE seizures. This sixteenth-century Spanish saint, also known as Teresa of Avila, founded an order of nuns and wrote extensively, producing an autobiography, three volumes of letters, and other books. One day while praying, Teresa reported, she "saw Christ close by me, or, to speak more correctly, felt Him; for I saw nothing with the eyes of the body, nothing with the eyes of the soul." Her confessor later asked her in what form Christ had appeared. "In no form," she replied.

Similar visions of Christ or God are common among Christian saints, many of whom developed a habit of mentally preparing for such visions. Brother Lawrence of the Resurrection, a seventeenth-century monk, wrote, "I know of one who, for forty years, has practiced the presence of God intellectually. . . . By repeated acts and by frequently recalling his mind to God he has developed such a habit that, so soon as he is free from external occupations," his soul "is lifted above all earthly things. . . . It is this which he calls the actual presence of God." This practice is thought to rely on developing mental control over patterns of charging neurons in the temporolimbic brain.

Kinsbourne does not consider all apparitions of the Virgin to be seizural, but another neurologist believes they are. Michael Persinger, a professor at Laurentian University in Ontario, Canada, has researched the neurophysiology of religious feelings and proposed that spiritual experiences come from altered electrical activity in the brain. If true, this would make religious experience a kind of TLE seizure. According to Persinger, religious and mystical experiences are "the *normal* consequences of spontaneous . . . stimulation of temporal lobe structures," which causes brain structures that are ordinarily unrelated to fire in tandem. The result is a mental experience in which unrelated states are linked. The person may have an early, perhaps infantile, memory of her parents and an out-of-body experience, which she interprets as a meeting with "God the Father." Or she may have auditory and visual hallucinations—"rushing sounds," voices, or "bright lights"—and a feeling of peacefulness, which her brain interprets as spiritual messages. In Persinger's view, religious experiences are our explanations for "microseizures," or "temporal lobe transients." He cited nonepileptic patients who have abnormal EEGs during religious experiences, such as a woman who spoke in tongues at her Pentecostal church and who, when she happened to speak that way at the hospital during an EEG, showed "spike-like events . . . from the temporal lobe."

Kinsbourne remains unconvinced that religious states and seizure states are frequently the same. "I don't believe [Persinger's theory], but I thought he was entitled to have his views published," Kinsbourne said. Cocking his head, he added, "It sounds insane, but it may turn out to be true."

Influential figures in three major monotheistic religions—Islam, Judaism, and Christianity—are thought by many to have had seizures. Scholars of medicine and literature have seen in Muhammad, for one, a possible case of TLE. "Muhammad assures us in his Koran that he had seen Paradise," Dostoevsky noted. "He did not lie. He had veritably been in Paradise in an attack of epilepsy, from which he suffered as I do."

A merchant and camel driver born in Mecca about A.D. 570, Muhammad had visions of angels who spoke to him for most of his life. Many of these recurrent visions occurred in caves in the mountains near Mecca, to which he, like other Arab men, often retreated for days or weeks of solitary fasting and meditation. At age forty, after having a series of strange dreams—bursts of brilliant light during sleep, which his wife felt made him even more shy and solitary than before—Muhammad withdrew to his cave on Mount Hara.

One night soon after his retreat, as he stood at the mouth of the cave, his mind suddenly lurched, according to the Koran. He felt himself being "seized" by a mighty external force that flung him to his knees. Something closed in on his senses, and he was caught in a vision like his dream visions, except that it could not exactly be seen. He sensed the presence of a "being," which he felt was Allah, or God.

The being ordered Muhammad to read the Arabic letters that had appeared before his eyes. "I do not know how to read," Muhammad protested. Again the being said in Arabic, "Read!" Muhammad felt oppressed, smothered, as if his breath were being squeezed from his chest. He felt he was about to die.

"READ!" the being commanded. "In the name of the Lord who created, who created man from a clot of blood. Read: In the name of a merciful Lord, who teaches by the pen, teaches men what they do not know." The being vanished, leaving Muhammad feeling as though these words had been inscribed on his heart.

Like a man possessed, he ran from the cave up the mountain toward a cliff from which he intended to jump. As he was climbing, the vision recurred. The dazzling figure of an angel appeared to him, a sight so awesome that he felt the urge to avert his eyes and avoid looking directly at it; but no matter where he turned, the bright vision was there.

"O Muhammad!" it said. "You are the Messenger of Allah, and I am his Angel Gabriel." Then the figure vanished.

Terrified, Muhammad ran the three miles home, threw himself down, trembling, and begged his wife to cover him, which she did.

After his fear had passed, Muhammad came to understand that he was being called as a prophet to preach God's word to the Arabs. For the next several years, he wandered through the nearby mountains, praying and attending to Gabriel's voice whenever it appeared. "Sometimes it comes to me like the reverberation of a bell, and that is the hardest on me; it leaves me when I have understood the message. And sometimes the angel takes the form of a man and speaks to me, and I understand

ıe says." At other times he heard a voice calling his name,
hen he turned to find its source, no one was there. Muham-
would panic, his heart would race, and perspiration would
ru down his face. Sometimes he felt bodily pain, or fell to the
ground, or had out-of-body experiences. In one such experience,
Gabriel led him to a huge, white steed that Muhammad mounted
and rode through the sky to Jerusalem, where he met Abraham,
Moses, and Jesus, drank some milk, and climbed Jacob's ladder
to God's throne in heaven.

Following these visions, Muhammad felt compelled to share
what they contained. Having convinced his wife and children of
the reality of his experiences, he began telling his friends, who
spread the word. His revelations, passed along orally at first,
were soon compiled by scribes in the Koran, the holy book of
Islam.

Muhammad also elicited skepticism. Christians, Jews, and
pagan Arabs jeered at him and called him insane. In 622 the ani-
mosity expressed itself in a plot against his life, which he discovered in time to escape. Under cover of night he fled Mecca and
went north to Medina, where the Islamic community solidified
around him. His army defeated armies from Mecca, and his
power grew. In his lifetime, his missionaries traveled as far as
Spain and Ethiopia, preaching his faith.

Muhammad's revelations, with their visual, auditory, and
emotional components, were not his only experiences that may
have been seizures. Legend has it that he was born with excess
fluid around his brain and that as a child he had fits. When he
was five years old, he reported to his foster parents, "Two men in
white raiment came and threw me down and opened up my belly
and searched inside for I don't know what." This might be a
child's interpretation of a seizure in which he sees flashes of
light, falls down, and feels abdominal pain.

To some observers, the possibility that neurological damage
underlies religious states such as Muhammad's discredits him
and diminishes their spiritual power. To others, this possibility
makes Muhammad's revelations no less expressive of truth than
Dostoevsky's novels or van Gogh's paintings. A few people have
even thought that the diagnosis of epilepsy enhances Muhammad's veracity and refutes the notion that he was insane. Certain

nineteenth-century commentators, for instance, in the throes of scientific positivism, considered the diagnosis of epilepsy proof of what Muhammad said, because while the voices of angels or God are not scientifically verifiable, seizural voices are.

"I am the God of your forefathers, of Abraham, of Isaac, and of Jacob," a voice said to Moses in about 1300 B.C. as he tended his father-in-law's flock on a mountainside in the Sinai peninsula. The voice seemed to come from an angel that appeared to Moses in the image of a burning bush. Though the bush seemed to be in flames, its form did not change. Like Muhammad with Gabriel, Moses was frightened by what he saw, and he hid his face.

In an extended dialogue that is recounted in the Old Testament, God commanded Moses to return to Egypt, where he had been born, to rescue the Jews from bondage and bring them to the Promised Land. Though fearful, the mystified shepherd followed the command. Setting out for Egypt with his wife and children, he again heard God's voice, telling him how to disarm the pharaoh. For years after leading the Jews back to Sinai, he heard the voice on the mountain. The recurrence of this experience suggests to David Bear that Moses had TLE.

Like Muhammad, Moses took on the role of God's spokesman, and he had difficulty convincing his people of the truth of what he had seen and heard. Once the Jews formed a community in Sinai, Moses told them of the God who appeared to him "in a thick cloud," with thunder, lightning, smoke, or trumpet blasts. He showed them the mountain and encouraged them to worship the new God there. During one forty-day period of prayer and fasting on the mountain, he heard the voice convey to him the Ten Commandments. Though he reported this message to his people, they remained uncertain of the new God. One day Moses came down from the mountain to find the Jews feasting and carousing in celebration of the old, pagan gods. In anger, he smashed the stone tablets on which he had inscribed the commandments, breaking the Jews' covenant with God. Later he renewed the covenant, returned to the mountain, rewrote the commandments on new tablets, and descended to his chastened followers. He died an old man, in eastern Sinai, on a mountaintop overlooking the Promised Land, to which his people, through his transforming experiences, had been called.

In the same part of the world more than thirteen centuries later, a young man rode toward Damascus. A Jewish Pharisee who held Roman citizenship, he had studied the Mosaic law in Jerusalem with a leading rabbi. Now he was on a mission. His purpose: to arrest and try followers of Jesus, the Jewish teacher who had been crucified in Jerusalem four years before. This man was one of the many who wanted to destroy the early Christians and their nascent faith.

Nearing Damascus, he saw a bright light flashing around him, and he fell to the ground. He heard a voice cry, "Saul, Saul, why are you persecuting me?"

"Who are you?" he wondered aloud.

"I am Jesus," the voice said. "Go into the city, where you will be told what you are to do."

Rising, Saul found that he was blind. A companion led him by the hand into Damascus. For three days he could neither eat nor drink, but then his sight returned ("it seemed that scales fell from his eyes"), his appetite returned, and he began to understand the meaning of this sudden, fateful event. A changed man, he was baptized, took the Roman form of his name, Paul, and became an apostle of Christ. His new mission: to spread Christ's message beyond the Jews to the Gentile world. He proclaimed Jesus the Messiah in the synagogues of Damascus, and he spent the rest of his life traveling throughout the Mediterranean region and the Middle East, preaching Christianity. His sense of personal destiny, like Moses' and Muhammad's, was strong.

Saint Paul's seizurelike experiences are the best documented of the major religious figures. His own numerous letters to the Galatians, the Philippians, and others compose a distinctive part of the New Testament. Paul's life story, including the conversion episode, is also told in the Acts of the Apostles, which was authored by a physician, the Gospel writer Luke, a sophisticated Greek who traveled with Paul. While Luke could not have known that epilepsy originated in the brain, he was familiar with its presentation, having mentioned a boy with grand mal seizures whom Jesus cured. Luke and Paul agreed that Paul suffered from an unknown "illness," or "bodily weakness," which Paul called his "thorn in the flesh." Biblical commentators speculate that this illness could have been migraine headaches or epilepsy. Migraines, thought to result from the expanding and shrinking of blood vessels to the brain, share symptoms with TLE, including nausea, numbness, and temporary speech difficulties. More common among epilepsy sufferers than in the general population, migraines on occasion respond well to treatment with anticonvulsant drugs. The "most natural hypothesis," according to the physician Albert Schweitzer, is "that Paul suffered from some kind of epileptiform [epilepsylike] attacks." Epilepsy could have resulted from malaria, which Paul is said to have had, and which involves a high fever that can damage the brain.

Paul's conversion experience strongly suggested TLE to David Landsborough, an English neurologist, who also cited "substantial" evidence that Paul's TLE seizures occasionally developed into secondary grand mal attacks. Landsborough considered Paul's sudden flash of light, his fall, the voice he heard, his temporary blindness and loss of appetite, and his abrupt recovery all consistent with a seizure, the blindness being a rare seizural aftereffect. The conversation between Paul and Jesus seemed to Landsborough to "represent an intensely vivid psychic aura," the state before a seizure, "engendered by Paul's thoughts and growing spiritual conviction during the preceding days. Epileptic experiences can be patterned by preexisting events, especially emotional ones."

Landsborough interpreted as a seizure another major episode in Paul's life, which is mentioned in a letter to the Corinthians. Writing about himself in the third person, Paul described an other-worldly trance that consisted of "visions and revelations," of being "caught up into the third heaven—in the body or out of the body, that I do not know," and of being "caught up into Paradise," where he "heard secret words that no human lips can repeat." Landsborough found in this trance the seizural features of ecstasy, a sense of unreality, or depersonalization, and auditory and visual hallucinations. Paul had other visions, often while praying, including one of a person begging for help and two of Jesus. Rather than dismissing his illness, Paul made it central to his mission. His account of his sufferings and ecstasies in his letter to the Corinthians ends, "Now I will most gladly boast of my weakness, that the power of Christ may dwell in me. Therefore I rejoice in weakness . . . and affliction for Christ's sake."

Landsborough believed that the diagnosis of epilepsy does not affect Paul's religious significance. "Natural events may influence individual decisions," the doctor wrote. "A cataclysmic natural event such as a first epileptic attack may have influenced Paul at a critical point in his thoughts. The incidence of such an event in his life does not diminish the reality of his spiritual change—from which he never wavered." There is no doubt that Paul stuck to his faith even as many clamored for his death. When he was about fifty, he was taken into custody in Jerusalem by the Romans, imprisoned for two years in Caesarea, and shipped back to Rome, where he was held under house arrest for at least two more years and beheaded in A.D. 67.

Long before Landsborough described Saint Paul as having had TLE, the psychologist William James mentioned the saint in arguing that religious states are in no way diminished by an association with abnormal mental states. "Even more perhaps than other kinds of genius," James wrote, "religious leaders have been subject to abnormal psychical visitations. Invariably they have been creatures of exalted emotional sensibility . . . liable to obsessions and fixed ideas; and frequently they have fallen into trances, heard voices, seen visions, and presented all sorts of peculiarities which are ordinarily classed as pathological. Often, moreover, these pathological features . . . have helped to give them their religious authority and influence," as in the case of Muhammad. "To plead the organic causation of a religious state of mind . . . in refutation of its claim to possess superior spiritual value, is quite illogical and arbitrary" because it implies that "none of our thoughts and feelings, not even our scientific doctrines, not even our *dis*-beliefs, could retain any value as revelations of the truth, for every one of them without exception flows from the state of the possessor's body at the time. . . . Saint Paul certainly had once an epileptoid [epilepsylike], if not an epileptic seizure"; but "how can such an existential account of facts of mental history decide . . . on their spiritual significance? . . . There is not a single one of our states of mind, high or low, healthy or morbid, that has not some organic process as its condition."

*   *   *

Sometimes a path to religion, seizures are also at times a path to art. Dostoevsky gave actual epilepsy to at least four of his characters, but most writers with TLE disguise their seizures in their work, using seizural experiences to lend emotional intensity to character or plot. One example is the French writer Flaubert, who had TLE seizures from age twenty-two until his death. Flaubert's typical seizure began with a feeling of impending doom, after which he felt his sense of self grow insecure, as if he had been transported into another dimension. He moaned, had a rush of memories, saw fiery hallucinations, foamed at the mouth, moved his right arm automatically, fell into a trance of about ten minutes, and vomited.

Flaubert gave features of these seizures to various characters, none described as epileptic. The heroine of *Madame Bovary*, unhappy with her husband, unable to pay mounting debts, and abandoned by her lovers, falls into a "stupor" while crossing a field near her home. The earth seems to yield beneath her feet. Strange memories crowd her mind. She fears she is becoming insane. "Suddenly it seemed to her that fiery spheres were exploding in the air like bullets when they strike, and were whirling. . . . They multiplied and drew near, they penetrated her. . . . She was panting as if her heart would burst." In an "ecstasy of heroism," she runs to the pharmacy, where she devours arsenic. Within days, she is dead.

Likewise, the title character in Flaubert's *The Temptation of Saint Anthony*, a hermit who lives in a desert hut by the Nile, hallucinates voices and visions. He feels the presence of "some monstrosity . . . floating around." In trances similar to Strieber's out-of-body experiences, he flies through space and time. Images flash before his eyes; he hears demons shriek; he becomes faint; "an unspeakable fear takes possession of him, and he feels nothing more of living sensation, save a burning contraction of the epigastrium. In spite of the tumult in his brain, he is aware of an enormous silence which separates him from the world." He cannot speak and "falls prostrate upon his mat."

Even "A Simple Heart," Flaubert's tale of the selfless maid-servant Félicité, contains a suggestion of epilepsy. While dying of pneumonia, Félicité watches, ecstatic, as her stuffed parrot, Loulou, seems to become the Holy Ghost. "She thought she could see, in the opening heavens, a gigantic parrot hovering above her head." Flaubert admitted to identifying with Félicité. While composing "A Simple Heart," he kept on his worktable a mounted Amazon parrot, borrowed from a museum in Rouen, much as his character keeps her beloved Loulou on the wall. And in his story she is struck down by a mail coach on the Honfleur road near Saint-Gratien, the very place where, in January 1844, the author suffered his first full seizure.

The twenty-two-year-old Flaubert and his brother were riding in a single-horse carriage on the road to Honfleur. As they neared the Saint-Gratien forest, Flaubert, who was holding the reins, suddenly fell back from his seat in a seizure that he later called an "excruciating snatching of the body from the soul." Lights flashed before his eyes. Flames seemed to engulf his body. An agonizing memory was unloosed in his mind. His brother, a doctor, drove him to a nearby house and bled him; bloodletting was then the only treatment for many illnesses, including epilepsy. When Flaubert regained consciousness, his brother drove him home to Rouen, where their father, a surgeon, diagnosed the attack as "epileptiform," a term that he, like many other doctors, considered less shameful than "epilepsy." The father based his diagnosis on Gustave's brief loss of consciousness, his visual and sensory hallucinations, and his vivid memory. A century later, doctors conjectured that Flaubert's complex seizure symptoms originated in the back of his left temporal lobe, as a result of brain damage in childhood or at birth. Flaubert had seizurelike experiences even as a child, sitting alone in a chair for hours staring into space and playing with a lock of hair or biting his tongue, then falling senseless to the floor.

Guy de Maupassant, the apprentice to Flaubert who became something of a son to the childless author, produced another literary description of seizures based on personal experience. Little is known about Maupassant's medical history except that as a youth he contracted syphilis, which damaged his brain, causing hallucinations and physical and emotional pains, and led to his death, at forty-three, in 1893. The neurologist William Gordon Lennox and other doctors regard as evidence of TLE Maupassant's short story "The Horla," a first-person account of a haunting.

The narrator starts out feverish, depressed, and fearful, overtaken by a "vague distress." He suffers an "attack of nerves" that afflicts both mind and body. "I have this constant, horrible feeling of a danger threatening, this apprehension of impending misfortune or approaching death . . . which means no doubt the inroads of some disease, unknown as yet." His doctor prescribes one of the earliest drug treatments for epilepsy, bromide of potassium, which provides no relief. The narrator becomes paranoid: overcome with dread, he repeatedly checks his locks and looks for intruders under his bed. He has trouble sleeping and, when asleep, is awoken by terrifying "seizures." He senses a presence nearby, "drawing close to me, looking at me, feeling me, . . . kneeling on my chest, taking my neck between his hands and squeezing, . . . trying to strangle me." In the garden a rose stem seems to break from its bush and rise in the air. He fears he is going mad. "Some unknown disturbance must have taken place in my brain," he concludes. "Is it not possible that one of the imperceptible keys of the instrument within my brain has refused to work?" What "if the faculty that records within me the unreality of certain delusions should be dormant just now?" He is convinced that his mind has been dominated and enslaved by a "mysterious will-power," which he calls "the Horla," or "my familiar." He decides to kill the Horla by setting him on fire. At the end, realizing that the Horla is still alive, within him, like a disorder of the mind, he resolves to kill himself.

TLE seizures may also be the source of events in the novels of Philip K. Dick, the twentieth-century visionary who published forty-one works of science fiction. The biographer Gregg Rickman has called TLE a "promising avenue for further research into the mystery of Phil Dick's experiences." From age fifteen Dick suffered from a recurrent ailment, never diagnosed, involving attacks of panic, fear, macropsia, micropsia, and depersonalization, as well as auditory and visual hallucinations that he interpreted as signs from God. This ailment brought on depression and suicide attempts and may have prefigured his late religious visions. Many of its symptoms found their way into Dick's books. In *Valis*, his 1981 cult novel, a character experiences the presence of God when "beam after beam of information-rich colored light" is fired into his brain, "right through his skull, blind-

ng" him and "imparting to him knowledge beyond
xperiences and even complete identities are elec-
ted into and retracted from human consciousness
emember It for You Wholesale," the story that
is for the film *Total Recall*. In *Do Androids Dream
, ...ric Sheep?*, the novel on which the film *Blade Runner* was
based, "Penfield mood organs"—fantastical machines no doubt
named for the surgeon who stimulated the brains of people with
TLE—induce in characters altered states of mind, such as
ecstasy, "awareness of the manifold possibilities open . . . in the
future," and despair.

TLE appears, too, in the works of the twentieth-century
American writer Walker Percy, whom Bear suspects of having
had the disorder. Percy trained as a psychiatrist at Columbia
University in the early 1940s, then converted to Roman Catholi-
cism and abandoned medicine in order to write. In his six novels
he attempted to "translate" his ideas about psychiatry and philosophy into the lives of characters in New Orleans, where he
lived. His heroes are typically depressed loners who are seen by
others as odd. In *The Thanatos Syndrome*, a Catholic priest has a
seizurelike "spell" that he describes as "not a dream but a complete return of an experience which was real in every detail—as
if I were experiencing it again, . . . captured in every detail, sight,
sound—even smell." The priest asks his psychiatrist, "Is there
something . . . which is not a dream or even a daydream but the
memory of an experience which is a thousand times more vivid
than a dream but which happens in broad daylight when you are
wide awake?"

"Yes," the doctor replies. "It could be a temporal-lobe
epilepsy—which often is accompanied by extraordinary hallucinations."

The central character in *The Second Coming*, another Percy
novel, experiences not only "temporal-lobe seizures" but also,
according to Bear, a disguised version of Geschwind's syndrome.
The character's recurrent seizures, which usually occur on the
golf course, involve visual hallucinations, funny smells, powerful
memories, and blacking out. He also experiences a general deepening of emotions—pronounced alterations in sexual interest, a
preoccupation with mysticism, prolonged depression, and "inappropriate longing" of a philosophical nature—which his doctor

identifies with seizures and calls "Hausmann's Syndrome." Bear, who noted while reading the novel that its style "is epileptic—slow-going and repetitive," wondered if these details arose from Percy's own life. Although he was never able to discuss TLE with Percy, who died in 1990, Bear did confront Percy's nephew, a doctor who practiced in Boston. "The nephew and I met somewhere," Bear said, "and I couldn't hold my tongue. I said, 'I'm just very curious about your uncle. I've read this book and it's about epilepsy. Does he have seizures?' 'I think so,' his nephew said."

The Victorian poet and dramatist Alfred Lord Tennyson also transformed suspected TLE seizures into art, but only after having been reassured that a seizure disorder was not what he had. As a young man, Tennyson learned that he had epilepsy from his doctor, who based the diagnosis on Tennyson's report of three childhood convulsions, on the "waking trances" that he had experienced regularly for several years, and on his family history. The occurrence of seizures is higher than normal among close relatives of epileptics, and the epileptics in Tennyson's family included his father, a paternal uncle, several brothers, a first cousin, and probably his paternal grandfather. The incidence of epilepsy in the family was probably even higher, since British doctors of that era saw masturbation as epilepsy's cause and were loathe to report its presence in respected families. The family also had psychiatric problems: Tennyson's father was alcoholic; two brothers were insane; a third brother was addicted to opium, and a fourth to alcohol; and the rest of his ten siblings suffered breakdowns. In 1809, as an infant, Tennyson himself had three convulsive seizures, after which he appeared dead. Repeated seizures in childhood can lead to adult epilepsy, especially TLE; in one study, one-third of the cases of TLE could be traced to severe convulsions before the age of five.

Tennyson's "waking trances" began in adolescence. Describing these mystic visions, he wrote, "All at once, out of the intensity of the consciousness of individuality, the individuality itself seemed to dissolve and fade away into boundless being; and this not a confused state, but the clearest of the clearest, the surest of the surest, the weirdest of the weirdest, utterly beyond words." In some trances "a great and sudden sadness would

come over me, and I would . . . wander away beneath the stars."
In London the image once came over him of "the *whole* of its
inhabitants lying horizontal a hundred years hence. . . . It was
not exactly a trance but the world seemed dead around and
myself only alive." He sensed that his mind had detached from
his body and his body was no longer his, which "might have
been the state described by Saint Paul, 'Whether in the body I
cannot tell; or whether out of the body I cannot tell.'" Tennyson
learned to bring on these mental states by silently repeating his
name.

Embarrassed by the diagnosis and its association with masturbation, Tennyson kept his seizures to himself. At thirty-nine,
he consulted a new doctor, who said his "fits" were not due to
inherited epilepsy but were instead the symptoms of gout, an
arthritic disorder that causes pains, fevers, and chills. This diagnosis released Tennyson from the humiliation of epilepsy,
enabling him to see his trances as innocuous, even illuminating.
As a consequence, he felt free to write of fits and trances in many
of the major poems of his middle age. In "The Ancient Sage," for
instance, he describes his own seizure state, depersonalization,
brought on by repeating his name:

> More than once when I
> Sat all alone, revolving in myself
> The word that is the symbol of myself,
> The mortal limit of the Self was loosed,
> And passed into the nameless, as a cloud
> Melts into heaven. I touched my limbs, the limbs
> Were strange, not mine—and yet no shade of doubt,
> But utter clearness, and thro' loss of Self
> The gain of such large life as matched with ours
> Were sun to spark—unshadowable in words,
> Themselves but shadows of a shadow-world.

Hidden or diagnosed, admitted or unknown, the mental
states that occur in TLE seizures are more than simply neurological symptoms. In people like Tennyson, Saint Paul, and van
Gogh, these states may have provided material for religion and
art. People with TLE, whether or not they know the physiological cause of their seizures, often incorporate their symptoms

into poems, stories, and myths. And the disorder does more than provide the stuff of religious experience and creative work. TLE is associated with personality change even when seizures are not occurring: it amplifies the very traits that draw people to religion and art.

CHAPTER FIVE

Personality

In an office at a veterans' hospital in Boston, amid makeshift ash-trays, sprawling cacti, and assorted images of owls, Edith Kaplan riffled through papers, pulled out drawers, and rummaged in files. A clinical researcher, she was searching for a drawing by one of her brain-damaged patients. "It's impossible to find anything in my office!" cried Kaplan, a short, stocky woman of sixty-four. Returning to her overladen desk, she shouted, "Here it is!" and raised a white page on which a patient had drawn a clock face. The clock face was octagonal, rather than circular. Arrayed within its precise double border were twelve neat numbers, for the hours, and sixty perfect tics, for the seconds. The clock's three hands—one more than most people draw—indicated a time of 11:10:32 o'clock. "Isn't it wonderful?" Kaplan exclaimed. "It's a temporal-lobe-epileptic clock!"

Drawing a clock face is one of the most common tests of brain function that neurologists give their patients. The test provides information about abstract thinking, language comprehension, memory, and even personality, and it is more revealing of the nature of brain damage than any other test known to Kaplan, whose field is neuropsychology, the study of the relationship between behavior and the brain. "If I have only *two* minutes with a patient," Kaplan said, "I ask him to draw a clock, put in all the numbers, and set the hands for ten after eleven." As the patient works, she watches the process, analyzing it and taking notes. Does he start on the right or left side of the page? Does he begin with the circle or the digits? Where does he place the hands? What, if anything, does he leave out? If he makes errors, does he appear to notice them? Is anything extraneous added? The drawing done, she deduces which parts of the patient's brain, if any, are damaged, and suggests a diagnosis.

A "normal subject," someone without brain damage, naturally draws a normal clock—a circle with twelve digits spaced uniformly, the hands at eleven and two. Most brain damaged patients draw clocks containing errors or lacking crucial parts. These mistakes depend on the kind and location of the patient's brain damage, so that the appearance of the clock face signifies what is wrong inside the brain.

Damage to one cerebral hemisphere produces predictable errors. Clocks drawn by patients with right-hemisphere damage usually contain errors of contour, while left-hemisphere damage usually produces errors of detail. This is further evidence of the right hemisphere's involvement in understanding the spatial whole, and the left hemisphere's control of parts, lists, numbers, and words. In a "right-hemisphere-damaged clock," as Kaplan calls it, the circle comprising the clock face is usually distorted or incomplete, and "nonverbal" features like the clock's hands are often left out. The numbers, which as "verbal" features are generated by the intact left hemisphere, are typically included, but they are often scattered because of the loss of spatial orientation. In some cases of right-hemisphere damage the entire left side of the page is blank because the patient is mentally blind to the left side of space.

As right-hemisphere damage impairs the drawing of the overall shape, left-hemisphere damage impairs the drawing of the details. Most left-hemisphere-damaged clocks contain a normal face with too few or no numbers for the hours. Some patients with left-hemisphere damage "overwrite," writing the same number repeatedly in the same spot, probably because of damage to the left frontal lobe, which regulates verbal behavior and enables a healthy person to cease one task and move on to another. Patients who have had strokes in the left temporoparietal region, controlling language and memory, may draw nothing because they cannot understand the instructions.

Like patients with unilateral brain damage, which is frequently the result of a stroke, patients with other neurological problems create clocks that are distinguished by whatever is omitted or awry. Patients with Parkinson's disease, a disorder of a lower brain region controlling basic movements, draw tiny clock faces with scrawled numbers that shrink as the patient writes. Remarkable effects appear in clocks drawn by people with Alzheimer's disease and other dementias that damage the frontal lobes, disrupting abstract thought. Asked to draw "ten after eleven," these patients typically place the hands on the clock at ten and eleven, failing to translate the number ten into "ten minutes" in order to set the minute hand at two. Kaplan attributes this error to the frontal-lobe damage that occurs gradually with age in everyone and rapidly in people with Alzheimer's. She calls this error "the frontal pull" because the patient is "pulled up or to the perceptual features of a task"—here, the literal, concrete ten—and thus makes "a stimulus-bound response," in which the stimulus, the number ten, is compelling in itself. This display of the frontal pull in drawings of "ten after eleven" assists in early diagnosis of Alzheimer's, which is why Kaplan prefers this test to "twenty after eight," the time that neurologists more commonly ask their patients to draw. "Twenty after eight" is not so effective in detecting frontal-lobe damage because, while it requires converting the word *twenty* into the numeral four on the clock, the lack of the number twenty on a clock face prevents a patient who might want to set one hand on twenty from making this stimulus-bound error. (But "ten after eleven" and "twenty after eight" are equally good for detecting damage in either cerebral hemisphere, because both require patients to put one hand on each side of the clock.) Many patients with frontal-lobe damage supply figures beyond the twelve usually found on a clock face, adding the numbers thirteen, fourteen, fifteen, and so on. Kaplan attributes this "perseveration" to the patient's tendency to be drawn to the digit sequence itself, which overrides his ability to remember he is drawing a clock.

People with TLE—in contrast to people with Alzheimer's, Parkinson's disease, and strokes—distort nothing, and they leave nothing out. In fact, their drawings of "ten after eleven" are more than correct; they are replete, displaying what Kaplan calls an "excessive, heightened attention to details." Another TLE clock that she found on her desk is as precise as the first; it has a brand name, "Westclox," at its center, and a winding pin emerging from its base. While some TLE patients produce ordinary clocks, most of their clocks are unusually detailed, unlike all the clocks of normal subjects and patients with other disorders. "When I get unusual clocks like these," Kaplan added, pointing to the two on her desk, "I know the person has TLE."

TLE clocks are "wonderful" to Kaplan because they elegantly demonstrate the direct relationship between brain activity and a personality trait. Brain changes determine the kind of clock the TLE patient draws. An epileptic scar in the emotional brain appears to overstimulate emotion-controlling tissues, causing patients to feel more deeply, so that even between seizures they display heightened attention to detail, a trait akin to the hypergraphia, hyperreligiosity, and stickiness that Geschwind found in his patients with TLE.

While Kaplan in her research was not looking specifically for objective corroboration of Geschwind's findings about links between personality and TLE—her main interests are disorders of language and movement—she was pleased to have found it in the TLE clocks. She had known Geschwind since the 1940s, when she was studying psychology at Brooklyn College and he was a premed student at Harvard, and they had worked together in the late 1950s and early 1960s at a Veterans Administration hospital in Boston. VA hospitals have been magnets for brain researchers since World War II, when many severely brain-damaged soldiers returned from combat. The patients at these hospitals include a high percentage of smokers, drinkers, and overweight people. These conditions in combination with serious brain damage tend to produce "advanced bread-and-butter pathology," such as strokes and epilepsy, the two most common neurological disorders, as well as other common conditions like Alzheimer's. In 1962 Geschwind and Kaplan collaborated on a landmark paper about the "split-brain effect," in

h brain hemisphere operates autonomously because
; cable that connects them is damaged. In their con-
about behavior and the brain, Geschwind and
en discussed the characteristic personalities of people with TLE.

Kaplan's TLE clocks demonstrate that, as Geschwind suspected, the links between personality and physiology encompass
talents as well as deficits. Unlike the clocks of patients with
strokes, Alzheimer's, and Parkinson's disease, TLE clocks are not
obviously disordered but instead show a heightened skill. While
many disorders illuminate the links between brain damage and
functional losses like neglect and distortion, TLE is unique in
showing that physical changes in the brain are related to functional advantages, too.

The biographies of famous people who are thought to have
had TLE contain numerous instances of the benefits of traits of
Geschwind's syndrome. The hypergraphia of van Gogh, Lewis
Carroll, and Dostoevsky is well documented. Tennyson, who
wrote voluminously from childhood, explained the pull of hypergraphia in the poem "In Memoriam":

> for the unquiet heart and brain,
> A use in measured language lies;
> The sad mechanic exercise,
> Like dull narcotics, numbing pain.

Philip K. Dick, who published his first short story at age thirteen, wrote "at white heat," according to biographer Lawrence
Sutin, and produced thousands of pages of handwritten journals
in addition to his many books.

Also known for his prolixity was Flaubert, who composed
essays and stories from the age of ten and kept a journal all his
life. "At the end of a day spent struggling over a few lines of his
novel-in-progress," the biographer Herbert Lottman observed,
"he could produce a considerable number of pages of correspon-
dence." In addition to extensive published fiction, Flaubert left
masses of drafts, unpublished writings, and lengthy letters. TLE
troubled him for most of his life, but it also excused him from
the profession of the law, to which his family had directed him.
"My illness," Flaubert confessed, "has given me the advantage of

spending my time as I wish." Writing was all that the reclusive Flaubert wished to do.

"Ten winged pens at once would not suffice!" Soren Kierkegaard said of his own compulsion to write. The Danish philosopher published many sermons and repetitious religious tracts and kept a daily journal from his youth. The psychiatrists Heidi and L. Bork Hansen find evidence of TLE in Kierkegaard's work and life. Soon after his death at age forty-two in 1855, a psychologist named Sibbern reported that the occasional paralysis experienced by the philosopher in his legs was "undoubtedly caused by epilepsy." A man who saw Kierkegaard regularly said he "often had excruciating attacks of his disease, during which he fell on the floor, but squeezing his hands and straining his muscles, he fought his pain and did continue the interrupted conversation, often saying: 'Do not tell anyone of this, there is no need to tell people what I am bearing.'"

Whether or not Kierkegaard was aware that these symptoms suggested epilepsy, he assiduously kept them secret "After my death," he wrote, "no one will find in my papers the slightest information (this is my consolation) about what really has filled my life." His story "Repetition," however, which the Hansens consider a veiled autobiography, contains passages about states of ecstasy moving to horror similar to the seizures described in Dostoevsky's *The Idiot*. "Precisely at one o'clock," Kierkegaard wrote, "I was at the highest peak and surmised the dizzy maximum which is not indicated on any scale of well-being, not even on the poetical thermometer. The body has lost all its earthly heaviness, it was as though I had no body," and "in that selfsame instant I toppled down almost into the abyss of despair." In his journal Kierkegaard confessed of suffering from a "disease" in which "the psychic and the somatic dialectically touch each other." Echoing Saint Paul, Kierkegaard called this disease a "thorn in the flesh," but said its anguish was indispensible to his productivity. "If my suffering, my frailty, were not the condition for my intellectual work," he wrote, "then of course I would still make an attempt to deal with it by an ordinary medical approach . . . but here is the secret: the significance of my life corresponds directly to my suffering." While the majority of writers with TLE are most productive in the periods when seizures are quiescent,

Kierkegaard may have been among the few who work best when seizures are occurring frequently. One such patient, a poet who was treated for TLE at Boston's Beth Israel Hospital, explained, "When my seizures are under control" with anti-convulsant drugs, "the muse leaves me."

The hemisphere in which epileptic activity occurs correlates with the nature of the resulting hypergraphia. In general, patients with epileptic activity in the left hemisphere write, and patients with right-brain epileptic activity engage in the plastic arts, such as drawing and sculpture. The reason, Kaplan said, is that left-sided scars overstimulate the left-hemisphere function of language, and right-sided scars enhance the visual-spatial skills led by the right hemisphere. These results are consistent with the errors in drawings of "ten after eleven" by patients with unilateral damage from strokes.

While most patients whom doctors describe as hypergraphic are writers, Bear studied four patients with right-hemisphere epileptic activity and consequent "visual-spatial hypergraphia." One was a successful potter, another a professional painter, the third an amateur poet-illustrator, and the fourth a quilter. Not surprisingly, all four patients displayed other aspects of Geschwind's syndrome. The potter was "sexually abstinent, pro-foundly religious, and intermittently aggressive," Bear said. She etched biblical quotations on every pot she made, to the dismay of her agent, who felt that the pots would sell better without spiritual messages. The work of the painter, which Bear saw as reflecting her "philosophical and spiritual questing," was com-pared by a critic to van Gogh's late work. The poet, a former nun, "developed multiple conflicts involving sexual preference, explosive temper, and . . . as her poetry turned increasingly to moral and religious themes, she began to incorporate apho-risms in brightly colored, extensively detailed drawings." And the quilter was "preoccupied, in a manner reminiscent of Dosto-evsky, by the question of whether religion was the highest achievement of mankind or a cruel instrument of social oppres-sion."

In an article about these artists, Bear theorized that visual-spatial hypergraphia occurs when epileptic activity in the tem-porolimbic region "tells" the frontal lobes, the decision-making part of the brain, "that many stimuli or events are salient—worthy of focused attention, novel, awesome, erotic, demanding explanation. The cumulation of such experiences may ... prompt prefrontal circuitry to initiate sincere moral or religious inquiries eventuating in artistic creations." While Kaplan circumspectly said that TLE enhances "productivity," Bear went further, calling the resulting work "creative." Citing van Gogh, Dostoevsky, Muhammad, Saint Paul, and Moses, he said that "a temporal lobe focus in the superior individual may spark an extraordinary search for that entity we alternately call truth or beauty."

Many people, doctors and patients alike, resist the notion that abnormally firing neurons can alter behavior and emotions—in positive or negative ways. As Spiers explained, "Who wants to think that a great literary work is based on a disease?" Yet the association between epilepsy and giftedness has long been noted. "Genius," wrote Cesare Lombroso, a physician of the nineteenth century, "is a symptom of hereditary degeneration of the epileptoid variety." While no one would call genius a "symptom" today, hypergraphia is acknowledged to be a product of the epileptic brain.

Hypergraphia may involve intensification of the feelings that lead anyone to write or draw. Kierkegaard suggested this when he called his disorder "the inscription on my innermost being that interprets everything and that often turns into events of prodigious importance to me that which the world would call bagatelles and what I regard as insignificant if I remove the secret note that interprets them." Similarly, hypergraphia may mimic the neurological process underlying the drive to create art. Certainly one purpose of art (and perhaps religion) is to reconstitute in words and images the structures and details of meaningful experiences that are gone, to remake the past, to stave off the loss of whatever felt beautiful or true. As Albert Camus said, an artist's work "is nothing but a long journey to recover through the detours of art the two or three simple and great images that first gained access to the heart." A general intensification of feeling and memory could certainly produce such a drive.

The similarities between the ongoing neural activity of a nonepileptic writer, artist, or religious leader and that of a person with TLE and Geschwind's syndrome remain unclear. In a study of ordinary patients at Beth Israel Hospital, doctors wrote, "The tendency or even compulsion to write excessively has been apparent in many TLE patients we follow, including some of the most well adapted and highly functioning. These patients may take creative writing courses, belong to poetry groups, or write short stories. Some of the work they produce is obsessive, ruminative, and moralistic; some of it, however, is poignant, insightful, and well written. It could certainly be argued that these patients do not differ from thousands of nonepileptic individuals who enjoy writing. However, it is the driven nature of the writing, its excessive quantity, and the repetitive moralistic and philosophic content that we tend to associate with TLE." Often, the doctors noted, hypergraphia seemed out of character when it appeared soon after patients developed TLE: a gym teacher with no previous intellectual interest suddenly became obsessed with writing something important; and a "semiliterate" laborer in his forties abruptly began recording his daily theological meditations. "In the hands of the untalented," as Geschwind put it, "the translation of the epileptic experience to the printed page fails to achieve literary greatness."

While hypergraphia and hyperreligiosity are often considered admirable, whether or not they produce great art, other traits of Geschwind's syndrome are not. To many people, increased aggression, altered sexuality, and even stickiness are socially unacceptable. As Charlie Higgins once said, "People who can't turn off the spigot are a pain in the neck." Yet these traits, too, are found in famous people with TLE. Moses, Flaubert, and Saint Paul were, like Dostoevsky, famous for their rages. Moses first departed Egypt for the Sinai to avoid being captured by authorities for having killed a man in anger; later, he smashed the tablets on which he had scratched God's commandments. Flaubert was "brutal," his mother said; a customs official nearly arrested him for assault. Saint Paul was a "relentless opponent," according to the historian C. H. Rieu, a "whirlwind of passions" in whom hate and depression merged with tenderness and love, "all in extremes." Prior to his conversion Paul was notorious for his thoroughness in persecuting Christians. The Gospel writer Luke captured Paul's stickiness: one evening in A.D. 58, while bidding farewell to his congregation in Corinth, Paul preached for so many hours that one listener went to sleep and fell from the window ledge where he was sitting. Paul revived the young man and returned to his speech, continuing until dawn.

Tennyson's irritability clashed with the same trait in other writers with TLE. He and Edward Lear, a shy, gentle painter and comic poet who had a seizure every day or two throughout his adult life, were close friends, although it is unlikely that either knew of the other's TLE. Lear, believing masturbation the cause of the disorder his doctor had diagnosed, struggled to conceal it for fear it would reveal the habit he had tried to break since adolescence. While visiting the Tennysons, in 1867, the future author of "The Owl and the Pussycat" offered to sell them some of his paintings. Tennyson fussed about the price, and Lear erupted in anger. He apologized that evening, but the two were never close again.

Extreme sensitivities caused the relationship between Tennyson and "Lewis Carroll" to end just as abruptly. Tennyson met the Reverend Dodgson in September 1857, when his wife, Emily, invited the minister to photograph her two small sons. Dodgson pronounced Lionel and Hallam Tennyson the most beautiful boys he had ever seen and produced portraits in which two blond, somber children recline awkwardly, wrapped in oriental cloaks. The boys apparently enjoyed the sessions, because Dodgson was asked back to take more pictures, including one of their father. Posing for his portrait, Tennyson, bearded and nearly fifty, sat stiffly in a chair against a flat background, his hat and manuscript pages in his hand. Later the two men corresponded, and Dodgson returned as a houseguest. In the late 1860s he wrote Tennyson asking permission to keep a privately printed copy of a song Tennyson had written and abandoned, refusing publication. The poet replied coldly, in a letter penned by his wife, "Dear Sir, A gentleman should understand that when an author does not give his works to the public he has his own reasons for it." Dodgson wrote back objecting to the implication that he was not a gentleman, to which Tennyson admitted in another letter that Dodgson had done nothing wrong. Dodgson responded, "You first do a man an injury, and then forgive him. . . . You first tread on his toes, and then beg him not to cry out." The friendship of two easily injured souls with TLE was at a close.

Sexually and interpersonally, all of these creative luminaries were distinguished by a combination of emotional intensity and restraint that is consistent with Geschwind's syndrome. Kierkegaard, who never married or had a known sexual relationship, considered sexuality an abomination, according to the Hansens. Saint Paul frequently recommended sexual abstinence, his own preferred state. In his first letter to the Corinthians he wrote, "To the unmarried I say: it is a good thing to stay as I am myself; but if they cannot control themselves, they should marry. Better to be married than to burn with vain desire." Paul was one of the few celibates among the leaders of the early Christian church, most of whom were accompanied on their missionary journeys by their wives. In an era when homosexuality was punishable by death, Paul may have been a repressed homosexual, according to John Shelby Spong, an Episcopal bishop. Spong based his theory on the saint's dislike of women, his never marrying, and his description of bodily torments. Among proponents of abstinence in the early church, Paul probably wrote and exhorted his readers the most, providing the foundation for the celibacy of the Catholic clergy.

Asexuality was also a prominent characteristic of Tennyson's. Robert Bernard Martin, a biographer, concluded that Tennyson was "not a deeply sexual man." His most important relationship was with a college classmate he knew from ages nineteen to twenty-three. The friend, Arthur Henry Hallam, whose age was the same as Tennyson's, died of a stroke caused by an undetected brain malformation, prompting Tennyson's poem "In Memoriam." "It would be hard to exaggerate the impact Hallam made on Tennyson," according to Martin, who considered the time of their friendship "the most emotionally intense period he ever knew, four years probably equal in psychic importance to the other seventy-nine of his life." Many women pursued the young Tennyson, but he was consistently uninterested. "There is not the slightest evidence that he ever had any sexual experience with another person until his marriage at the age of forty-one," Martin wrote, and Tennyson said "he had not so much as kissed a woman" until the year he married. His thirty-seven-year old bride was a semi-invalid, already confined by a spinal problem to a couch for most of each day. Despite great affection and the birth of two sons, the marriage was not passionate; soon after the wedding the Tennysons began sleeping apart.

Flaubert was similarly withdrawn and intense. The French writer spent his adult life in his childhood home, living first with his mother, until her death in 1872 when he was fifty, and then with his beloved niece. His close relationships outside the family were carried on largely through letters. His appetite for sex was ordinary or even excessive when he was a teenager, but it diminished abruptly and dramatically at the time of his first seizure. Before his seizures started, he had visited prostitutes regularly. Afterward, he became an ascetic, eschewing all sexual activity for more than a year. "Humping has nothing more to teach me," Flaubert told a friend at twenty-three. "My desire is too universal, too permanent, and too intense for me to have [physical] desires." Later, he developed homosexual interests. "While he was quite capable of an affair with a woman, particularly a somewhat distant one," the biographer Benjamin Bart wrote, "his real interest, his affection and, one may even say, his real love went to" men. He joked in letters to close male friends about being homosexual, and mentioned having sex with men in the Cairo public baths. He wrote of wishing he were a woman, and sometimes dressed in women's clothes. His famous love affair with Louise Colet involved little face-to-face contact; he wrote her scores of letters but refused to allow her to come to his house. Despite her pleading, he never considered marriage.

Flaubert's temper, stickiness, and altered sexuality did not prevent him from functioning at the highest level in his art. In fact, Geschwind's syndrome apparently contributed to his accomplishments, lending a passionate focus to his personality and his work. In ordinary people, however, the syndrome may not be so beneficial. Kaplan recalled one TLE patient at the VA hospital with a "flagrant, indisputable" case of the syndrome whose "heightened sense of the meaning and importance of everything" compelled him to complain to a supermarket manager that the cans on the store's shelves were not arranged alphabetically. When the manager refused to rectify the situation, the man become so critical and moralistic that the manager threw him out of the store. The patient wrote frequent letters to editors and to utility companies, complaining about seeming errors in the newspaper or in his bills. Keith Edwards, who was a resident in neurology under Geschwind's supervision in the early 1970s, recalled one TLE patient of Geschwind's who was "fanatically religious and wrote all sorts of things for hours at a time. This man was obsessed—controlled, almost—by an omen or sense of doom."

In Gloria Johnson, an unusually magnified version of Geschwind's syndrome has produced a social outcast. Highly sexed, compelled to write, and intensely moral and emotional, Gloria in her youth and early adulthood committed several violent crimes, for which she served time in jail. Her ability to express her rage through violence has been hampered since her early forties by rheumatoid arthritis. Yet at fifty-nine she remains quick to anger, a trait that she channels into civic activism. Unable to move about easily, she sits and awaits news of societal ills beside her phone, which on account of her clinginess, persistence, and moral outrage is a formidable tool.

Not long ago, someone left a garbled message on her telephone answering machine that sounded to her like "You nigger! You black!" Gloria discovered this message when she returned to her apartment from a public celebration at Boston City Hall, to which Geraldine Cuddyer, a mayoral aide, had invited her. Cuddyer and other public functionaries whom Gloria calls with her complaints occasionally invite her to such events, hoping that she will feel appreciated and thus cause fewer problems on the phone. Gloria had had a nice time at city hall—Cuddyer's secretaries had given her a cake in honor of her birthday—but her mood changed when she heard the message. She suspected someone working at city hall had left it, although she did not know who.

Outraged, she sent a telegram to the mayor. She left messages for Cuddyer and for Richard Jones, a press secretary for the mayor, saying she wanted to discuss racial discrimination at city hall. The next morning, she phoned the bishop, played the message for him, and said excitedly, "That's not right. They called me 'nigger.'" The bishop soon ended the conversation by asking her, as usual, to pray for him. "Thank you, Bishop Riley, I will," she said, and they both hung up. Then, irritated by the city's lack of response to her calls, she decided to complain in person at city hall. "I wanna fight!" she said, not uncharacteristically.

She called the office of Geraldine Cuddyer to warn her that she was on her way. The secretary said Cuddyer was out to lunch. Gloria erupted, "Damn, they always say that," slammed down the phone, and dialed again. When another secretary said Cuddyer was at a meeting, Gloria barked, "Well you tell her I need to talk to her." She hung up and said pleasantly, "She's nice, that one is." Her irritation returning, she added, "But they're putting me off. When the doctors do that, at least they come out in the open!" Gloria has switched from doctor to doctor over the years in an effort to find those who give her adequate telephone time. Now, her anger renewed, she packed a shopping bag with her purse and the documents that she considers her tickets to power—letters from powerful people she has known, including clergymen, doctors, and public officials—and arranged for a friend to drive her back downtown.

As she waited for an elevator in the city hall lobby, she reflected on her mission. "There are two mayors in this city," she announced grandly to a crowd of strangers, "but I'm the main one. He's the white Irish mayor," she explained, referring to Boston Mayor Raymond Flynn, "and I'm the black West Indian mayor!" When the elevator came, she parked her wheelchair in the rear and demanded quiet. "I run this place," she continued, turning to the distinguished white-haired man standing next to her. He ignored her, but others peeked past him to see who was making the fuss. They saw a sixtyish woman in a wheelchair, wearing a white polyester sweater, green slacks, Bradlees running shoes with lacy white socks, and numerous bracelets and rings. Her short, dark hair was disheveled. Protective braces encased her ankles and wrists, and a collar support encircled her neck. She clutched the plastic shopping bag on her lap.

No one had responded to Gloria's remarks, so she tried again. "The mayor's got his whole family working in here," she said. "He's a crook." A few people laughed. Encouraged, she continued, "I'm handicapped. I want my cut. I want my slice of the pie!" There was more laughter; the crowd was amused. This pleased Gloria. The emotional intensity resulting from her temporal-lobe damage causes an inordinate desire to be liked and appreciated, but it also compels her to stir things up. In addition, suspected frontal-lobe damage reduces her inhibition about saying whatever comes to mind.

The elevator stopped at the floor occupied by the mayor, and Gloria's companion rolled her out. As they exited, Gloria smelled something odd and pungent, like whiskey; this was a seizure symptom. "Who's been drinking?" she demanded, staring accusingly at the white-haired man. It is not clear if she was actually seizing; her seizures and her personality bleed into each other, making it hard to say where one ends and the other begins. Some of her seizures involve confusion, tears, anger, and fear. However, seizing or not, she is emotionally labile. The traits of Geschwind's syndrome are present all the time.

Minutes later, Gloria remembered which door led to the office of the mayor's immediate staff. She rolled herself into the suite, greeted by name the first secretary she saw, and suddenly began to shout. "This is Mrs. Johnson speaking! Open these doors! No racial discrimination!" Rolling herself past the secretary, she entered the office marked GERALDINE CUDDYER.

Cuddyer was standing at her desk. When she raised her eyes and saw Gloria, she looked stunned. While she had invited Gloria here the day before, with ample notification to the security staff, Cuddyer was disturbed that Gloria had returned on her own. "What are you doing here?" she demanded.

"I wanted to see you," Gloria pleaded.

"You should have called."

"I *did*, Gerry." Gloria pouted. "I called you a hundred times. Every time they say you're busy."

"I am busy," Cuddyer affirmed. "What's this about?"

"I'm very upset," Gloria said, like a child who has finally gotten a parent's ear.

"Look, Gloria, we had a nice visit yesterday," Cuddyer said, hoping to remove the intruder as quickly as possible. She knew from experience not to say anything that might provoke Gloria's anger. She said blandly, "You and I sat here and had a nice little chat."

"Yeah, but see," Gloria replied, her volume increasing,

"there's racial discrimination in here. And this is supposed to be the city of Boston, where *everybody is treated fair.*"

"Don't shout," Cuddyer said quietly. She thought for a moment, aiming to avoid a confrontation. "I don't know, Gloria," she conceded, her voice laced with fatigue. She determined not to disagree openly with Gloria. As hard as it is for most people to decelerate a heartfelt argument, it's even harder for Gloria, who lacks the normal emotional controls. Just as TLE seizures intermittently abolish free will, Geschwind's syndrome continually reduces free will, so that a person with TLE is no more in charge of her moods than of her seizures. People who understand this are more successful in dealing with Gloria than people who don't.

Unprovoked, Gloria had calmed down. "I'm too upset," she acknowledged quietly. But then, recalling the answering-machine message, she cried, "I am an epileptic, and for some reason someone called me a nigger on my phone." Cuddyer wisely said nothing, and Gloria decided to go. She would take her complaint to Richard Jones, the press secretary who had not responded to her calls. Rolling herself away from Cuddyer, she said, "I'm concerned about the city tactics, and what's going on between white and black!"

"I'm sorry you feel we have to have an altercation," Cuddyer said. "Go home, and have a happy birthday." She closed her door the moment Gloria was outside. Gloria rolled herself out of the suite, muttering to the secretaries, "Racial discrimination is real bad around here." Returning to the elevator, she asked someone to help her get to the mayor's press office. One floor up, a blue-suited woman who worked in the building entered the elevator and greeted Gloria warmly. "I was here yesterday," Gloria said proudly.

"Two days in a row!" the woman replied supportively.

Turning sullen, Gloria said, "I got mistreated."

"I can't believe that!" the woman said, concerned. "Who mistreated you?"

"Gerry Cuddyer."

"Not Gerry. She'd never mistreat you. She thinks you're the best." Without condescending to Gloria, she had disagreed with her. Flattery often diverts Gloria's anger.

The woman accompanied Gloria into the press room, where she introduced her to several city hall employees who seemed pleased to meet the person who pestered them on the phone. Someone remembered her birthday, and they all shook her hand and wished her well. "Thank you, darlings," she said, thrilled. When not threatened, Gloria can be ebullient; her emotional lability has positive effects. A tall man in a seersucker suit glided by, and Gloria said to the crowd, "I think I cussed him out one time."

"Probably," someone replied. "You've cussed out most of us. How come you never apologize?"

"I'm sorry, everybody!" Gloria said joyfully, laughing from the gut. Doctors have observed that, unlike sociopaths, most people with TLE genuinely feel sorry for their antisocial acts.

Just then, Gloria remembered why she had come. "I want Richard Jones!" she cried. Someone left and returned with Jones, a tightly wound man in his thirties who seemed less sensitive than Cuddyer and the friendly woman on the elevator to Gloria's limitations. Instead of greeting her warmly, he held himself aloof. When she snarled at him, he snarled back, apparently unaware that provocation is her way of warming up to people, that her behavior is largely out of her control, and that she reacts poorly to treatment like her own.

For the next hour, in a private office to which Jones took her to discuss her "allegations of discrimination," they engaged in a heated verbal battle. She recited her credentials, foremost among them her six years of "lecturing" at Harvard Medical School.

"Harvard Medical?" he broke in, incredulous.

"I have letters to prove it," she snapped back. "I'll show you," she said, shuffling through the worn envelopes in the bag on her lap for the thank-you letters that Bear sent her each year after her visit to his class. Jones refused to look at them, which angered her more.

In dealing with Gloria's impassioned complaints, Jones made several tactical mistakes. He ignored her pleas for sympathy. Each time she calmed down, he failed to take advantage of it, proposing instead to refute her allegations with facts, which fueled her emotional fires. In their ensuing shouting match, he raised the heat further by suggesting that she might file a class action suit against the city, to which she replied, "Yes, I will," although the idea had never crossed her mind. He suggested she was lying, which set off another litany of complaints. As she searched frantically through her purse and among the letters that were now on the floor for one from Bishop Riley, Jones told her, "Don't drop this stuff all over."

"Watch it, honey," she warned. She threw him a killing look and began another diatribe about racial discrimination, the rights of the handicapped, and housing problems. Her ire now unleashed, she used profanities, to which she resorts when all else has failed. Interrupting her, he charged her with being difficult and unkind, and she countered, "I'm *real*, honey. I'm *me*." She had a point. She is unexpurgated, without restraint. The person on whom all of this is hardest is Gloria herself, who has to live with it full time.

Finally, Jones tried to make a joke: "You didn't bring the posse in here, did you?" Gloria's anger climaxed in a rush of words, as her sneakers bounced on the foot flaps of her wheelchair. Realizing that she could become physically violent, she growled to her companion, "Let's go, before I punch him out. I don't wanna hurt him." She grabbed the wheels of her chair and turned herself around, preparing to leave. Jones taunted her, "Time to go?" prompting her to spin around and unleash yet another torrent of rage. She emitted low, hostile, inarticulate sounds, and spit at him.

He seemed shocked. "I tried to help you out," he said.

"No, honey," she warned, "I don't need no help from you. The mayor needs help from *me*!" Noticing a heavy glass ashtray on the desk beside her wheelchair, she grabbed it and shook it. "Nobody likes to hear the truth, do they?" she shouted. "But my Bible tells me, Jesus said the truth will set you free. Jesus was not a liar! So you better not put your praying hands together and take no eucharist if you don't believe what Jesus said was true!" Her face wrinkled with disgust. She brandished the ashtray and threatened, "You want me to hit you?"

Twenty years earlier, a neurosurgeon who had been her doctor told her to stay away from people who bother or irritate her. "That doctor told the truth," she conceded on a calmer afternoon. "I asked him why he said that, and he told me, 'Because something triggers off in your brain.' I said, 'What is it, a gun?'

He said, 'On that order.' And he was right. I can go off just like that."

Jones grabbed the ashtray from Gloria and growled, "Don't you dare hit me." Suddenly she looked bewildered and dazed. She let out a little sob.

Just then a security guard whom Jones had alerted during a quick telephone call quietly entered the room. "I'm Tim from Security," the burly young man said, shaking her hand. "I'm the one you like, I think," he added hopefully. He asked her how she was. She smiled and chatted amiably. Tim posed no threat; he wasn't challenging her. Jones silently left the room.

The next minute, she scowled and turned her irritation on Tim, complaining that the lining of his pants pocket was exposed. "That reminds me, my father used to do that," she said. She told him to straighten his tie, which he attempted, looking like a boy on his way to a prom. Still Gloria wasn't satisfied. He advised her to try to relax. As they talked, he pushed her chair out of the office and across the lobby. "Hold that elevator!" she cried to a stranger. Looking wasted and puffy, she boarded it and moaned, "I don't feel right. Nothing's right. I feel bad. I'm ready for bed."

In the car on the way home, she was quiet, thinking about the traits that motivate her to fight city hall. She caught sight of a torn chain-link fence surrounding an abandoned lot, which gave her an idea. "There's links in city hall like in that chain over there on that fence," she said, pointing to the fence. "There's always a link somewhere that needs to be fixed. It's broken, and *I* have to fix it." Indeed, more than most people, she is troubled by the broken links in fences. Sticky, hyperreligious, and grandiose, she has trouble giving up. Something compels her to try to fix things, to right wrongs. That something, according to Bear, is the electrical activity underlying TLE, which makes her as zealous in pursuit of a vision of justice as was Saint Paul.

The negative associations of increased anger and altered sexuality cause doctors to disagree about the presence of Geschwind's syndrome in ordinary patients. While a highly sexed person like Gloria with a history of violence is viewed as an obvious case, high-functioning TLE patients who behave appropriately in meetings with their doctors are sometimes said not to have the syndrome. When the traits appear more subtly than in Gloria, Flaubert, or van Gogh—especially when a patient's emotions are reduced rather than intensified—doctors have difficulty detecting the syndrome. Because it can be manifested in opposite ways, it can be difficult to detect.

Some neurologists consider Geschwind's syndrome questionable—even pernicious—as a diagnostic category, and therefore prefer not to look for it out of regard for their patients with TLE. The neurologist Thomas Browne said that the risk of further prejudicing the public against epileptics is greater than the benefits of publicizing the syndrome, which "puts an additional burden on people who already have enough trouble getting along in society." The president of the Epilepsy Foundation of America, according to Bear, "has publicly denied the connection between TLE and personality in an attempt to protect people with epilepsy from discrimination, while he privately told me that he knows the syndrome exists." Most neurologists who oppose publicizing the syndrome consider its traits negative: it is a "personality *disorder*," the neurologist David Coulter said, "a cluster of pejorative attributes, which gives people with epilepsy a bad name." Just as some doctors refuse to use the word *epilepsy* with patients because of its negative associations, doctors who consider the traits negative do not discuss Geschwind's syndrome with patients.

Charlie's neurologist is one of those who don't ask about the traits. A slight man with a blond goatee, Edwards sees roughly three thousand patients a year from Vermont, western Massachusetts, and central New York, about three hundred of whom have TLE, grand mal epilepsy, or both. During his residency in Boston, Edwards met Geschwind—"a genius of the caliber of Einstein; I listened to his weekly teaching rounds and hung around him every chance I got"—and a few of Geschwind's patients with TLE. The younger doctor's impression was that "the patients with the syndrome were *odd*, to use a nonmedical term. I mean, if you met one of them on the street, you'd know there was something a little wrong with them; they were almost schizophreniclike, except they were more personable, with better peer relations, than schizophrenics. Most of my patients with TLE today are nothing like that."

Edwards offered his patient Charlie Higgins as an example.

Having defined the traits as "pathological," the doctor was compelled to say that someone as well-adjusted and little impaired by TLE as Charlie cannot have them. Although Charlie had expressed his concern to Edwards about losing "libido" and becoming "excessively verbal and detailed," the doctor maintained that "Charlie's personality has not been affected by his TLE or the underlying brain scar." Thinking a moment, he added, "Oh, if there are studies that correlate TLE with obsessive personality, that would fit Charlie. He's a careful person, compulsive, a hard taskmaster on himself, overly focused. He thinks about some things so intently that sometimes he's just not listening. But I don't think his obsessiveness is a problem. He's not obsessive in a pathological way." Yet focused and obsessive thinking is associated with Geschwind's syndrome, according to Bear. Geschwind emphasized that the traits need not be "pathological" but can be found in anyone, ordinary or "odd." And Edwards himself, describing Geschwind's patients with the syndrome, used the word *obsessed*.

In many cases, the syndrome is not obvious. Pierre Gloor, a neurologist at the Montreal Neurological Institute, said that Geschwind's syndrome "hits you in the eye in only about ten percent of cases [of TLE], but that doesn't mean it doesn't exist in a somewhat hidden form in other patients. Sometimes you have to dig for it" by asking questions and paying attention to patients' interest in religion and sex. "If you don't look for it," Gloor added, "it won't show up."

If Edwards examined Charlie's personality, he would find nearly a mirror image of Gloria's emotionality. While Gloria is more illustrative of the syndrome because of the frontal-lobe damage that intensifies the syndrome's effects, Charlie is actually more typical. As Bear explained, "Most people with TLE express their strong feelings less flagrantly than Gloria does"; like Charlie, "they are far more circumspect." Absentminded and calm, Charlie displays intense but channeled aggression, reduced sexuality, moral fervor, and a compulsion for details. These traits are consistent with abnormal brain activity caused by the scar that he is suspected of having developed at age twelve. Geschwind's theory that personality change is caused not by TLE seizures but by the underlying scar may explain how in Charlie the syndrome could have preceded his seizures by thirty years.

While Gloria acts out her aggression by shouting obscenities and arming herself with broken bottles and knives, Charlie has found socially acceptable outlets for his aggression. "In the courtroom when I was trying cases," he said, "if I felt I knew the law better than my opponent, I was a little scornful of him, a little arrogant. A couple of times as a judge I got angered by the behavior of some of the lawyers and put them down pretty hard." More noteworthy than this professional snubbing is Charlie's dedicated daily run of several miles, which is motivated by his desire to release aggression. "Sports are the one place in society where aggression is acceptable," he explained, "just part of the game." He started running as a "painfully shy" seventeen-year-old, too small for football, who was allowed to join the track team. He was a competitive long-distance runner at Princeton, and even at age seventy he runs three miles a day.

Charlie displays a global reduction of interest in sex consistent with temporolimbic damage. His interest in sex diminished after his diagnosis, but it was apparently never strong even before. He was known around town as a prude. His minister recalled Charlie's plea for donations for a new church organ. "Whenever Charlie stands," the minister said, "people listen. Well, he got to talking about this new *organ*, and people started laughing and making double entendres. The more he talked, the more embarrassed he got, and the funnier it got for us. In all his propriety, Charlie was digging the hole deeper the more he tried to get out of it!" Within Charlie's family, his son, Michael, said, "there's a standing joke that Mom and Dad commemorated their two lovemaking experiences with babies." There was little physical affection between the parents, and no talk of sex between father and son. Even now, when Michael, a tall, athletic man with a family of his own, arrives at home and hugs his father, Charlie holds back, his arms at his side. "Sexuality is a subject I'd rather not get into," Charlie has said testily. "I'm of the generation that didn't believe in it—in talking about it, I mean."

Charlie's most prominent trait is his extraordinary calm. He speaks quietly and moves as if in a trance. People describe him as steady, even-handed, and controlled. Possessed of an almost angelic detachment, he seems serene, above the fray, so placid and still that in certain poses, as in his yard, wearing his weathered weekend clothes, he resembles a scarecrow. "He's absent-minded," his wife said; this trait goes back at least to his early twenties, when she met him. He tends to forget names. When he is driving she often has to remind him that a traffic light has turned green. If she isn't around, a driver behind him generally honks. According to his daughter, "if two cars simultaneously come to a fork in the road, Dad *always* lets the other car go, even if he's in a hurry, which he never is anyway." Fran added, "He's always been a daydreamer, low-geared. He always took his time doing things, and he was never easily alarmed. When he occasionally lost his temper, it was very mild; he never stomps around." Charlie's son added, "There was never any violence at home. We were always taught to turn the other cheek." Michael and Rachel each recall their father becoming openly angry only once. When they were small children, Rachel said, Charlie spanked them after finding them on a dirt pile that he had forbidden them to climb. A few years later, Michael, who was ten years old at the time, heard his parents "yelling just a little" in the kitchen. "I went in to them and said, 'Dad, you always tell me and Rachel that if we could only see ourselves fighting, we'd see how stupid we look. I'll say the same to you.' They stopped fighting right away."

"I don't have a genius for friendship," Charlie conceded, adding that he spends most evenings quietly at home. "He could be perfectly happy," Fran said, "just sitting reading all day." His daughter, a neurologist who has studied Geschwind's syndrome, observed, "He's passive overall, and I wonder if his epilepsy made him that way. It's like he's in that seizure state all the time." His lack of emotional intensity may indeed have a physical basis. His pulse is slow, always under sixty beats per minute, and his blood pressure is very low, usually 100/50. Since heart rate is regulated by temporolimbic structures, which also participate in emotions, there may be a connection between the damage to his temporolimbic brain and his slow heartbeat and emotional placidity—a version, perhaps, of Geschwind's syndrome.

Just as Charlie's overall calm seems rooted in brain activity, so does his limited obsessiveness, which, as he told Edwards, has increased since his diagnosis. Abnormal electrical activity in his left hemisphere may disrupt his overall concentration, causing his general absentmindedness, while it overstimulates other regions in the same hemisphere, causing his intellectual focus. This effect explains his paradoxical duality—how his mind can be pinned on an inner thought, while he remains emotionally detached and vague, unaware of the peopled world outside. Despite his absentmindedness, Charlie has a striking ability to focus on the details of philosophy, logic, the law, music, and nature. "He's talky," his wife noted. "If he has a captive audience and a subject he's interested in, there goes your day." Back from an African safari, he wanted to show his family five hours of videos he had taken of the flowers, animals, and birds that the entire family had seen. Fran pestered him for weeks to reduce the show to two hours and, eventually, to one. In conversations that interest him, he moves smoothly from one subject to another; practically anything reminds him of something he knows. Midstory, like a gifted child on show, he is both in a world of his own, unmindful of the listener, and conscious of performing, alert to holding the floor. His verbal segues—"um," "of course," and "on the other hand"—prevent listeners from politely breaking in. His preference for logic over emotion is even reflected in his work, in which he increasingly handles only legal research, leaving the interactive side of the practice, such as litigation and divorce work, to his partners.

Charlie's greatest obsession is religion. Since high school, when he often asked his teachers' permission to recite antiwar poems by Siegfried Sassoon and Rupert Brooke, he has had "a romantic sense of death" that found expression in a fascination with people who have gone to the edge, risking humiliation and even death for their beliefs. His heroes include Socrates, Albert Schweitzer, and Saint Francis of Assisi. "There is a strong element of self-denial characteristic of all of them," he explained. Having become interested in the writings of Socrates in college, Charlie took his interest farther than most casual readers. In his thirties he searched out *The Death of Socrates*, an academic study of the philosopher by a Roman Catholic priest named Romano Guardini, which still rests on his bedside table and to this day is his favorite book. "It's one of those things you can read over and over again," Charlie marveled. Indeed, he has read it thirty or forty times, underlining sentences and penciling remarks—"IMMORTALITY," or "DANGERS OF PLATONIC THOUGHT"—on its pages. As a young adult, Charlie also read Chesterton's biography of Saint Francis and Schweitzer's many books on theology, and often listened to recordings of the missionary doctor performing the organ preludes of Bach.

Charlie attended church services for the first time in the spring of 1942, while in Washington, D.C., on a training assignment for the Navy. He was first drawn to the Washington cathedral by the music of the organ and the choir, but his interest increasingly had a strong emotional element. Since then, he has maintained a close affiliation with his local Congregational Church, where he attends weekly services, often without his wife. He also participates in theological discussion groups, which leave him frustrated by the church's spiritual life; he wishes others were more interested in talking about religion. Even his minister, he complained, is not drawn to conversations about theology. To make up for this lack, Charlie talks religion with Catholic friends and reads extensively in the field. He prefers modern, liberal, largely Catholic theologians and disdains fundamentalism, which he considers overly emotional and intellectually unsound.

"I guess anyone could gather from my bookshelves," he said one day, with a shy smile, "that I'm interested in theology." His book collection, organized by category on shelves covering two large walls of his house, is heavy on philosophy and theology. There are six translations of the Bible, numerous biblical commentaries, and several books on worship or prayer. Charlie has sixteen books by C. S. Lewis and twelve by Albert Schweitzer, including *The Quest for the Historical Jesus*, *The Mysticism of Paul the Apostle*, and *Paul and His Interpretations*. The shelves contain *Early Christian Creeds* and *Early Christian Doctrines*, by J. N. D. Kelly, Maritain's *Reflections on America*, Pascal's *Pensées*, Augustine's *Confessions* and *The City of God*, and a multivolume study of the Reformation. Among the other titles are *My God and My All*, *The Candle of the Lord*, *The Faith of a Heretic*, and Thomas Merton's *The New Man*, as well as various works by the theologians Küng, Neibuhr, and Tillich. In all, this theology collection is equal to that of a well-stocked village library.

Charlie's mind moves naturally to theological subjects. One bright autumn afternoon, as he drove to his office from his weekly lunch at the Rotary Club, he was deep in thought on the subject of death. He remembered how odd it seemed that he didn't react with fear when in 1975 his TLE was diagnosed, a tumor was suspected, and he was faced with the possibility of imminent death. "I realized, of course, that anybody's death hurts others who are left behind, but I was not afraid. I wondered, Is there something wrong with me that I am so indifferent? How can I be so composed about my own final illness?"

He pulled into the driveway of his office building and conceded, "I'm not so sure how I'd do with suffering pain, if that were involved." He stopped the car. "I guess only God can suffer *all* the pain in the world," he mused. "Perhaps He saved the rest of us from suffering the pain of others, no matter how sympathetic we may be . . . " He raised the emergency brake lever. "Sometimes I'm convinced there *is* a life after death, and sometimes I'm not. The Jewish people had magnificent faith for millennia before they even started *thinking* about life after death." Charlie opened the car door an inch, but made no move to get out. He does this at home, too, if he is with anyone willing to listen to him in a stationary car.

"I have an inherent objection," Charlie continued, "to the idea of the quid pro quo of heaven as a reward for good behavior." He was silent for a moment, staring out the front window of his car. "Theologically speaking," he resumed, using a favorite expression, "the thought of nothingness doesn't appall me, because the uniqueness of one's personality is so intimately bound up with our sense of consciousness"; that is, a person experiencing nothingness would be unaware of it. "When theology speaks of people being raised from the dead following the Second Coming, what happens meanwhile?" he wondered. "It's a problem. I mean, if you're asleep for a thousand years, during which time you have no sense of being yourself because you're asleep, and suddenly you come to life again at the Second Coming, what's the difference between being asleep for a thousand years or for infinity?" Expressionless, he emerged from his car, walked up the path, and climbed the stairs to the porch.

"I think we have an instinctive fear of death, just as animal creatures do." He stopped on the porch. "Animals don't have a sense of death in the abstract, but they have an instinctive fear of what ultimately threatens them. We're animals, too." He chuckled and looked absently across the street, hands in the pockets of his raincoat. Just then, the outer door of the office building opened, and a client of Charlie's partner emerged. Charlie said hello automatically and entered the building.

Not surprisingly, Charlie's neurologist knows nothing about his religious life. "If Charlie is religious," Edwards said, "it's just part of his background. For a lawyer and an educated man, an interest in theology doesn't stick out." Yet Charlie was not raised in a religious family. Neither of his parents ever attended church or showed any interest in it, nor have his children, making this an unusual feature of his personality.

Charlie displays other aspects of hyperreligiosity. He is a strongly ethical man with a fine-tuned sense of justice. "He's the most honest person around," his son said, "the fairest I've ever met." If his moral outrage is aroused, this ordinarily passive man can be provoked to anger. One fall afternoon, as Charlie was raking outside his house, a gang of boys came onto the lawn and kicked apart a pile of leaves that he and Fran had amassed near the road. Charlie knew the boys were having a great time, but he also knew that what they were doing was wrong.

Charlie walked toward the boys, most of whom ran away, except one boy, twelve or thirteen years old, who stood, frozen on the grass. Ready to offer a quiet lecture on the privacy of lawns, Charlie approached the boy, who suddenly turned and bolted down the road. Charlie set off in pursuit. The boy didn't know that Charlie could outrun many youths.

At the end of the road, the boy made a mistake. He turned onto a lane that loops through the valley, returning to where it starts and offering no cover of woods. Charlie knew there was no escaping him now. He increased his pace. This would be his daily run.

The boy, surprised at Charlie's endurance, tried to run faster, so Charlie ran faster, too. Exhausted, the boy finally slowed. Charlie sped up and tackled him. "You're going to come with me," he ordered, "and rake those leaves back up in a pile." The boy followed and did what he was told. "He had to," Charlie said later, proud of having taught him a lesson.

In remonstrating against those who do injustice, Charlie is

like Gloria at city hall. While he would no sooner shout or swear than disrobe in public, he finds acceptable ways of expressing his moral outrage, stickiness, and unusual concern for right and wrong, applying his fervor and circumstantiality in ways that give him public credit rather than shame. The very traits that at one time made Gloria a prison inmate and mental-hospital patient contribute, in different combination, to Charlie's gifts, making him a pillar of his community. Her irritating persistence is a magnified version of his quiet determination. While tempestuousness and robust sexuality make her odd, muted anger and lessened sexual interest make him appropriate. In both Charlie and Gloria, it is the temporolimbic function of emotion that is altered from the norm. In her the TLE traits are mostly intensified, while in him all but hyperreligiosity are diminished. Abnormal electrical activity in the temporolimbic brain often has opposite effects—intensifying traits in one person, and decreasing the same traits in someone else.

Taken together, Charlie and Gloria demonstrate Geschwind's theory that the syndrome is intrinsically neither positive nor negative. The traits appear subtly and beneficially in Charlie. He makes no waves, does what is expected, and is, in short, an exemplary citizen: thorough, pious; self-controlled, patient, focused, and firm. Gloria, on the other hand, sticks out as "abnormal," like the "odd" patients Edwards remembered Geschwind presenting at hospital rounds. Yet Gloria and Charlie harbor the same peculiar disorder, and many of her feelings and reactions are as understandable as his. Some of her crazy seeming traits are exaggerations of his sane traits, such as awareness, compassion, and sensitivity. Her ideas and beliefs are reasonable; only their intensity is bizarre. Charlie's ideas and beliefs are reasonable, too; their intensity is unusually reduced. The brain abnormality that these two TLE patients share turns her emotional faucets up to full force and his emotional faucets down low, making her "odd" and him exceedingly "normal."

The TLE traits are variations of traits that appear in everyone, much as TLE seizures are variations of ordinary mental states. Most of us display a few traits of the personality disorders outlined in psychiatric manuals, and one or two of the TLE traits. Geschwind's syndrome can in fact be "more extreme in the normal individual than in the temporal-lobe epileptic," according to Bear, who, the first time he heard of Geschwind's syndrome, saw it in himself. While he was a student at Harvard Medical School in the late 1960s, Bear heard Geschwind lecture on the strikingly high incidence of certain traits in TLE patients. Reflecting on his own fascination with writing, religion, and philosophy, Bear, an intense young man who had graduated first in his class from Harvard College, immediately thought, "Gee, *I* have some of those characteristics!" After medical school, Bear went on to make the association between personality and TLE one of the theoretical pillars of his career, becoming the standard-bearer for Geschwind's syndrome after Geschwind's death.

"We *all* have these traits!" Bear said of Geschwind's syndrome, explaining that in everyone, personality is defined by brain events. Neural networks underlie our sexual interest, our aggression, and our interest in religion. Neural systems enable us to make emotional associations, telling us what is awesome, sexually arousing, and frightening. "This process goes on in all of us, in our temporolimbic regions, whether we're cool as cucumbers or tempestuous," Bear said. Other factors, such as experience, moderate the process: "whether our parents say, 'Don't take anything seriously,' or they are professional worriers, saying, 'Everything's a big deal,' influences the circuits, too." The difference between people with TLE and everyone else is that their brain lesions tend to push them a little further to emotional extremes. The disorder influences certain brain networks in predictable ways, altering the amplitude of emotions, leading to characteristic behavioral change. "When we talk about this behavior syndrome," Bear affirmed, "we're really not talking about bad things. It's a distortion that people with TLE are crazy or sex perverts or violent"; the vast majority of them are not. TLE is an illness "that affects the process of making emotions, bringing out some of the most magnificent and specially human behaviors," such as our excursions into morality, writing, and art.

The ordinariness of the traits makes them difficult to define. No one has quantified how religious, sexual, or aggressive most people are, so no one knows how much of any of these traits is "normal." Personality is largely subjective. None of Geschwind's efforts to find objective correlates of personality—such as asking

patients to count their sexual encounters or religious obser-
vances, weighing their written responses to a query about their
health, or noting how often they return to or phone a doctor's
office—solved the problem of determining the presence of
Geschwind's syndrome in an individual. Most doctors who
detect the traits in patients say they have a "feel" for them.
Schomer looks not for specific traits but for an overall emotional
change, and he relies on context: while frequent church attendance would indicate hyperreligiosity in someone from a nonre-
ligious family, it is the norm for a devout family; conversely, in
someone from a strongly religious background hyperreligiosity
might appear as deeply felt atheism.

These definitional problems cause disagreements among
doctors about the syndrome's prevalence. No hard figures exist,
and estimates vary. Thomas Browne, a neurologist who opposes
publicizing the syndrome, said it occurs in a minority of his
patients with TLE—by his estimate, 5 to 30 percent—while Bear
believes the syndrome "could be very common." Defining the
syndrome as two or three of the traits appearing together, Bear
finds it in a large percentage of his TLE patients, many of whom
are referred to him specifically because of his interest in personality. A group of researchers at Beth Israel Hospital concluded
that "one or more of these traits are frequently seen" in TLE
patients, "sometimes to a dramatic extent."

Bear, believing that the syndrome holds clues to the physical
bases of personality in everyone, has long sought objective criteria for determining the prevalence of the TLE traits. He and a
colleague took an important step in this direction in 1977 when
they formulated a "quantitative analysis" of personality with
TLE. To determine the extent to which these traits are present
in patients, Bear and Paul Fedio, a psychologist at the National
Institutes of Health, devised a questionnaire in which patients
could respond "true" or "false" to statements that tested for the
traits. Having determined that the traits were more subtle and
specific than the five that Geschwind identified—hypergraphia,
hyperreligiosity, stickiness, aggression, and altered sexuality—
Bear and Fedio added thirteen more traits: elation, sadness,
anger, guilt, emotionality ("deepening of all emotions"), hypermoralism ("attention to rules with inability to distinguish significant from minor infractions"), obsessionalism ("compulsive

attention to detail"), circumstantiality ("loquacious, pedantic, overly detailed"), viscosity ("tendency to repetition"), sense of personal destiny ("events given highly charged significance, divine guidance ascribed to many features of patient's life"), dependence, humorlessness, and paranoia. The questionnaire consisted of a hundred statements—five statements that tested for each of these eighteen traits and ten unrelated control statements. "I would like to write a book about my life" and "It makes good sense to keep a detailed diary" tested for hypergraphia. A "true" response to "I would go out of the way to make sure the law is followed" indicated hypermoralism. "Powerful forces are acting through me" tested for grandiosity and hyperreligiosity. Humorlessness was detected with "Few things are really funny," and statements such as "Things which never attracted me before have become sexually appealing" and "My sexual activity has decreased" tested for altered sexuality. For stickiness: "Once I start to talk to someone, I have trouble breaking off." And for aggression: "I would like to rip some people to shreds."

Bear and Fedio gave this questionnaire to twenty-seven people with TLE and twenty-one controls. The controls included nine people with unrelated neurological disorders and twelve people with no neurological problems. The researchers also gave the questionnaire to someone who knew each subject, usually a spouse or close friend, to determine if the subjects deceived themselves about their personalities.

In the responses of both the subjects and their acquaintances, the normal subjects rated lowest on Bear and Fedio's eighteen traits; the people with neurological disorders other than TLE rated slightly higher; and the TLE patients rated significantly higher than all of the controls in all eighteen traits. Bear and Fedio concluded that a smaller group of these traits suggested a basis for identifying people with TLE. "A consistent profile of changes in behavior (obsessionalism, circumstantiality), thought (religious and philosophical interest), and affect (anger, emotionality, and sadness) . . . appears to be the specific consequence of a temporal epileptic focus." TLE patients emphasized their own humorless sobriety, dependence, circumstantiality, and personal destiny, while people who knew them described them as obsessional, circumstantial, dependent, and sad. While none of the twenty-one controls had high ratings on these traits, all but one of the twenty-seven TLE patients had high ratings on them all. Consequently, positive questionnaire responses to these eight traits seemed a possible tool for diagnosing TLE.

The doctors also found a correlation between the location of the epileptic activity and certain traits: the traits clustered differently, depending on which temporal lobe contained epileptic activity. In general, people with right-hemisphere epileptic scars were excessively "emotional" and denied their unusual behavior and traits, while those with left-sided lesions were more likely "ideational"—sober, highly moral intellectuals who regularly scrutinized themselves and overemphasized their own abnormalities. Bear and Fedio speculated that this affect-thought dichotomy—another version of the right-left differences that Kaplan noted in drawings of "ten after eleven" and Bear noted in hypergraphia—results from overstimulation of one hemisphere, which enhances its functions.

Bear and Fedio's finding of a hemispheric effect on personality may explain the different displays of the TLE traits in Charlie and Gloria, and it may even suggest the location of the epileptic lesion hidden in Charlie's brain. "Emotional" describes Gloria, who indeed has a right-sided lesion, probably several. The scholarly, ruminative Charlie, on the other hand, neatly fits under the rubric "ideational." Although his doctors have so far been unable to pinpoint his lesion, his personality indicates that his lesion is in his left hemisphere.

Bear and Fedio's study has been partly discounted, on the grounds that their statistics are flawed. Their questionnaire lacks "negative questions," to which "false" rather than "true" would indicate the syndrome's presence (negative questions prevent subjects from figuring out the "right" answers from the questions' general drift). Moreover, Bear and Fedio did not test control groups with other affective, or emotional, disorders, such as depression and manic-depressive illness, whose personalities may not differ significantly from those of people with TLE. It is clear that some of the traits of Geschwind's syndrome are not unique to TLE. People with manic-depressive illness have a high incidence of hypergraphia. Repeated use of LSD or cocaine produces several of the syndrome traits. LSD alters tem-

function, perhaps by means of a mechanism similar
TLE, Bear surmised, causing people to become reli-
ilosophical, hyposexual, fearful, and paranoid; the
syndrome is a cousin of Geschwind's. Bear would like
the personalities of people before and after they use
LSD, but the illegality of the substance prevents such research.
The "best experiment" Bear can think of for studying the syndrome's frequency would be to assess the "change in emotionality" of a person before and after developing TLE; this is of course
impractical, since it is difficult, if not impossible, to predict who
will develop epilepsy. Kaplan thought of comparing the personalities of TLE patients both on and off anticonvulsant drug treatment, to discern the correlation between seizure frequency and
personality, but this study is also impossible, because doctors
cannot ethically withhold treatment.

The results of attempts to replicate Bear and Fedio's findings
have been inconsistent. In one study using the questionnaire,
psychiatrically hospitalized patients with TLE consistently
scored differently from nonepileptic psychiatric patients. In
another study, however, nonepileptic psychiatric patients were
almost indistinguishable from TLE patients. Questioning the
validity of the second study, Kaplan suggested that the
nonepileptic psychiatric patients who displayed the syndrome
may have had undiagnosed TLE: "To the doctors who argue that
they can go into any psychiatric hospital and find ten patients
with exactly the same thing [as Geschwind's syndrome], I'd say,
'How do you know those patients don't have TLE?'" The neurologist Shahram Khoshbin studied twelve such patients—psychiatric patients with Geschwind's syndrome but no evidence of
seizures—and found abnormal electrical activity in the temporal
lobes of all twelve. This abnormality, discerned on a computerized electroencephalogram known as a brain electrical activity
rapid display, or BEARD, was somewhat different from that
appearing with TLE. Khoshbin tried switching these patients
from antipsychotic drugs to anticonvulsants, with the result that
Geschwind's syndrome lessened in some cases. This surprised
the neurologist, since treatment of TLE with anticonvulsants
usually has no affect on personality. These studies raise as many
questions as they resolve; the exact relationship between person-

ality and seizures remains unclear. Despite these questions, most doctors concede that TLE is associated with emotional and personality change, and that the nature of the change is determined, as Bear and Fedio showed, by the hemisphere in which the epileptic scar is located.

In fact, Geschwind's syndrome now functions as a diagnostic tool. The syndrome may even be a better indicator of TLE than a clinical seizure or the EEG, because the traits are constant, while the seizures are abrupt and occasional, occurring only once a week or several times a day. "I'd trust the behavior over the EEG," Kaplan stated, "since the EEG may be negative because it's sampling at a time of quiescence"—that is, when the person is not seizing.

In some TLE patients, one striking personality trait clinches the diagnosis. Several years ago, a retired bank president came to Bear after being diagnosed with panic disorder and manic-depressive illness. An "ultra-high achiever" who had undergone a long but unsuccessful psychotherapy, the man listed various complaints. He described periodic panic attacks and spells in which his body seemed to change shape and he felt he was walking on his knees. Sometimes he lost his sense of where he was in space; once he blacked out on a train. He had a nasty temper: trivial details pushed him to rage. Twice divorced, he felt lonely and depressed. The seizure symptoms, extreme anger, and depression suggested undiagnosed TLE to Bear, but not until he heard the patient's "terrible secret" was the diagnosis made. "Sometimes I dress in women's clothes," the man confessed. In Bear's mind, suddenly "it all fell into place." The man's cross dressing, which seemed out of character in someone so conventional, and his temper were aspects of Geschwind's syndrome; his dissociation, blacking out, and panic attacks were seizures. An EEG turned out to be abnormal, confirming Bear's diagnosis. The man was prescribed anticonvulsant drugs, which calmed his spirits and reduced his strange sensations. When some time later he told Bear that, never having written before, he was now working on an autobiographical novel, the doctor was not surprised. "Although the disorder has not prevented him from functioning in a superior way," Bear said, "his personality has surely been influenced by epilepsy."

Whenever the syndrome is present, according to Bear, TLE may reasonably be considered as a possible cause. In 1986 the psychiatrist used the Bear-Fedio questionnaire to determine posthumously whether the author of *The Inman Diary*, a 155-volume, seventeen-million word memoir, had TLE.

Arthur Crew Inman was a native of Atlanta who, following a physical and emotional breakdown in 1916, at the age of twenty-one, left college and retired to a darkened, soundproof suite of apartments in Boston. Bedridden for the most part, he was attended by servants, physicians, and strangers whom he paid to talk to him. An inheritance supported this life-style. He complained of crippling aches and pains, visual and auditory hallucinations, and despair over the state of the world. He recorded these complaints and much more in a diary that he kept daily for more than forty years. He attempted suicide several times and in 1963, driven wild by noise from the construction of Boston's first skyscraper, he succeeded by shooting himself.

When Inman's lengthy diary was published in a two-volume abridgment in 1985, doctors and reviewers wondered if he had suffered from an undiagnosed illness. A medical report appended to the published diary suggests that the 1916 breakdown could have resulted from a viral infection, such as mononucleosis. But since no fever was reported, a virus was unlikely to have been present. Inman's unusual sensitivity to light and sound, as well as his hallucinations, suggested to both Bear and Shahram Khoshbin that Inman had migraine headaches. But migraines alone could not have accounted for Inman's unusual personality. TLE, these doctors agreed, was a more promising possibility.

The diary at least suggested that Inman had Geschwind's syndrome. To verify this possibility, two Bear-Fedio questionnaires were filled out separately for Inman by Bear and an editor of the diary, based on their familiarity with the diary's contents. The editor, Libby Smith, who had spent seven years reviewing the unabridged diary and interviewing scores of people who knew its author, had never heard of TLE or Geschwind's syndrome. Both she and Bear gave Inman high marks in all the TLE traits except "religiosity." "Compulsive attention to detail" described Inman's need to make lists and keep rigid schedules.

His childlike charm and tendency to fly into rages translated into high scores in several categories: "dependence," "deepening of all emotions," "humorlessness," "anger," and "paranoia." His effort to chronicle his era demonstrated his "grandiosity" and "sense of personal destiny." Overall, Inman scored substantially higher than the control groups and well within the range of people with TLE.

The personality syndrome could explain many of Inman's peculiarities, which bewildered his diary's readers. A story recounted by the osteopath who treated him for twenty-five years reads like a textbook definition of stickiness. "I would be sailing off Cape Cod," the osteopath recalls. "The Coast Guard cutter would come up. They'd say they had just had a flash that Arthur Inman wanted to see me immediately. I'd have to call him, ship-to-shore, and tell him I couldn't come right away. He'd say, 'You have to come.' I'd tell him it would cost him a lot of money. He'd say, 'I don't care. Just come.'"

The syndrome would also explain why sex held an intellectual fascination for Inman—why he liked to lie naked in bed with women and hear them describe their sexual feelings to him, but he disliked sexual intercourse and rarely engaged in it. "Inman must have had some kind of temporal-lobe or limbic disorder," Spiers said, "because he was both detached and intense, emotionally not connected to the world."

The presence of Geschwind's syndrome alone, however, is not sufficient grounds for diagnosing TLE. Confirmation of the diagnosis depends on the evidence of a brain lesion or an actual seizure state. Inman never had an EEG, and his scanty hospital records and autopsy report are unrevealing, so it is impossible to know if he had a scar in his brain. It may be relevant that he was addicted to two drugs used as anticonvulsants, potassium bromide and barbiturates, the latter of which is still regarded as effective in treating epilepsy. More important, his diary offers evidence of seizures. To Bear, Inman's description of his 1916 breakdown, which involved bizarre sensory and emotional states, culminating in an attack while he was at the home of friends, sounds like a TLE seizure. "My whole nervous system went on strike," Inman wrote. "Specks of light zigzagged in front of me. My ears whistled. . . . The room began to circle with a

·y motion, very bewildering. I heard them talking,
ons, but my ears were full of noise, and I could not
ìuddenly . . . I began to cry long, racking sobs, with-
ˈ After lying down for a while, Inman was able to
ʌds.

Other events described in his diary also suggest that he had
seizures. In 1919 he wrote of recurrent sensory and auditory hallucinations: "I feel as though I were undergoing a change such as
occurs in a violin string when the pitch is raised. This condition
has occurred to me time after time." Thirty years later he
lamented his extreme sensitivity to noise and light, which is consistent with TLE. "I live in a box where the camera shutter is out
of order and the filter doesn't work and the film is oversensitive,
and whatever that is beautiful or lovely registers painfully or
askew," he wrote. "The simplest factors of existence, sunlight
and sound, uneven surfaces, moderate distances, transgress my
ineffective barriers and raid the very inner keep of my broken
fortifications, so that there exists no sanctuary or fastness to
which I can withdraw my sensitivity, neither awake nor asleep."
Based on these apparent seizure states and Inman's personality,
Bear and Khoshbin concluded that the diarist had undiagnosed
TLE.

The nineteenth-century American poet and horror writer
Edgar Allan Poe also had Geschwind's syndrome without a diagnosis of TLE. Poe was obsessed with philosophy, phrenology,
and mysticism. He had a bad temper and stormy relationships.
At twenty-seven Poe married his cousin Virginia Clemm, a girl of
thirteen. After Virginia died, eleven years later, he remained
devoted to her memory, never marrying again. Biographers suggest that their childless marriage was never consummated. Poe
began writing in adolescence and was prolific, producing sixty-
eight stories and many other works, most considered too frantic
to be first rate. Ornate and digressive, his writings contain
lengthy descriptions of the habits of albatrosses, ways to trim
the sails of whaling ships, and attempts to reach the South Pole.
These works, like the man himself, demonstrate features of
Geschwind's syndrome. Fights, beatings, accidental deaths, mur-
ders, and suicides are general in Poe's tales. A critic observed
that "there is simply no sex in his writings." The women in his
stories, rarely described, are neurasthenic or dreamlike. Many of

his central male characters write extensively, are profoundly dependent on one other person, and are drawn to mysticism and philosophy.

In addition to these personality features, there are numerous seizurelike states in Poe's writing. Roderick Usher, a paranoid, sticky, hypergraphic, hyperreligious, and apparently asexual character in "The Fall of the House of Usher," suffers from a strange "madness," an "acute bodily illness," and is attended by a physician. Like Inman, he is extremely sensitive to light and sound, keeps his house dark, and lives isolated from the world. He has a weak stomach, physical pains, and a "nervous agitation." Often he feels powerfully afraid. He gazes "upon vacancy for long hours, in an attitude of the profoundest attention, as if listening to some imaginary sound." And the narrator, after arriving at Usher's house, suffers similar feelings of "gloom" and an "utter depression of the soul," like "the after-dream of the reveller upon opium." Objects look strange: the house seems to have eyes. He has a *déjà vu*: the unfamiliar house seems familiar. He develops an "irrepressible tremor" and suffers attacks of pain and fear. As he leaves the Usher house, he experiences visual and auditory hallucinations—a flash of light and a "long tumultuous shouting sound like the voice of a thousand waters"—and he feels that his brain has "reeled."

Similarly, in Poe's novel *The Narrative of A. Gordon Pym*, written when he was twenty-seven, several characters experience seizurelike disturbances of body and mind. The narrator, Arthur Gordon Pym, awakens "strangely confused in mind." His head "ached excessively"; he "fancied he drew every breath with difficulty"; he was "oppressed with a multitude of gloomy feelings," including "extreme horror and dismay." He falls into a stupor, a "state bordering on insensibility," and loses track of time. While climbing down the wall of a chasm, Pym experiences classic TLE seizure states—the sensation of falling, powerful emotions, a vision of a phantom, and the feeling of falling into the phantom's arms: "[I] at length arrived at that . . . fearful . . . crisis in which we begin to anticipate the feelings with which we *shall* fall—to picture to ourselves the sickness, and dizziness, and the last struggle, and the half swoon, and the final bitterness of the rushing and headlong descent. . . . There was a ringing in my ears, and I said, 'This is my knell of death!' . . . For one moment my fingers clutched convulsively upon their hold . . . in the next my whole soul was pervaded with a *longing* to fall. . . . I let go at once my grasp upon the peg, and . . . remained tottering for an instant. . . . But now there came a spinning of the brain; a shrill-sounding and phantom voice screamed within my ears; a dusky, fiendish, and filmy figure stood immediately beneath me; and, sighing, I sunk down with a bursting heart, and plunged within its arms." Throughout the novel, characters suddenly and for no apparent reason burst into tears and then abruptly fall asleep, as some people do after seizing. There is no pathos to these tears; they are overly intense and unmotivated, more typical of seizures than of grief. Despite the horror and other extreme emotions expressed throughout Poe's writings, there is little genuine feeling of an ordinary sort. "We are never admitted to the private recesses of Pym's own mind," a critic, Edward H. Davidson, noted. "We are always outside, in an external . . . representation of . . . inner states of being." The many acts of violence upon which so many of Poe's plots turn seem gratuitous; like seizures, they are sudden, shocking parodies of ordinary experience.

Poe in fact suffered from a mysterious neurological condition that was never diagnosed but is consistent with TLE. A "nervous sensibility" made him unusually sensitive to drugs and alcohol. As an adult in the 1840s he had major episodes of "delirium" in which he wandered city streets, muttered senselessly, perspired, and fell into unconsciousness, his limbs trembling; these may have been partial seizures that generalized into grand mal attacks. Perhaps his horror stories, which are replete with strange, terrifying happenings and characters haunted by ominous visions and sounds, vague illnesses, "nervous afflictions," and varieties of "madness," described his own experiences of bizarre sensations that he could not control. The disorder could explain not only these images and events but also the feverishness with which he wrote. As Geschwind said of Dostoevsky, TLE could have given Poe "a shortcut to apprehension of depth of emotion not readily available" to most people.

If Poe were alive today and diagnosed with and treated for TLE, he would probably still be driven to write. The current treatment of choice, anticonvulsant drugs developed in recent decades, is thought to have little or no effect on the personality syndrome. Even when the drugs succeed in reducing the number of seizures a patient has, her personality usually remains intact; in the infrequent cases in which drugs halt seizures altogether, the syndrome may intensify. Whether or not this presents a problem depends on the nature of the individual's traits. In Gloria and others in whom, according to Bear, the syndrome is "even more incapacitating than the seizures," controlling the seizures with drugs "often doesn't improve the patient's situation that much." But if the syndrome is innocuous, as in Charlie, or prodigious, as in van Gogh, Dostoevsky, and perhaps Poe, its removal could be a loss.

CHAPTER SIX

Intervention

In their attempts to relieve their suffering, Flaubert, Tennyson, and van Gogh all avoided the most painful nineteenth-century "cures" for TLE. These so-called remedies included prolonged application of a hot iron to the head or chest, intended to free the invading spirits believed to be the disorder's cause, and castration or clitoridectomy, which were thought to work by ending masturbation. Yet each of these artists had his share of ineffective treatments. Flaubert and van Gogh both took pills of potassium bromide, later discontinued as an anticonvulsant. All three submitted to hydrotherapy, or "the water cure," which was believed, erroneously, to minimize the effects of nervous disorders. A doctor ordered van Gogh to spend countless hours in tubs at the asylum in Saint-Rémy. At European spas recommended for epilepsy by Tennyson's doctor, the poet submitted to drinking large amounts of water, walking long distances in bad weather, and being plunged, wrapped in sheets, into cold baths. Still his trances did not cease. In 1844, soon after Flaubert's diagnosis, his father, a doctor, ordered him to take numerous baths and also prescribed herbal teas, infusions of orange blossoms, and regular bleedings with leeches. A few months later, Flaubert abandoned these useless, if standard, treatments and resigned himself to live with his affliction.

Today, although a host of newer treatment methods have replaced bleedings, hot irons, and hydrotherapy, for many patients the results have not changed dramatically. Alone among epilepsies, TLE does not respond particularly well to the anticonvulsant drugs that are now the first line of treatment offered for epilepsy. While 75 to 90 percent of patients with grand mal seizures achieve good seizure control with anticonvulsant drugs, less than 35 percent of TLE patients say that anticonvulsants control their seizures well; Charlie is in the lucky minority, while Jill and Gloria are among the other two-thirds. The reason for the different responses of generalized and partial seizures to these drugs is not clear, in part because doctors understand little about how the drugs work. Most anticonvulsants do not affect the seizures' source, the epileptic scar, but instead alter the surrounding biochemical environment, somehow blocking neurons in or near the scar from spreading epileptic activity and thus raising the brain's seizure threshold.

Drugs are used first for TLE because they are the easiest and least invasive form of treatment. The first few years after a diagnosis with TLE are often spent trying various drugs, to find out which, if any, work. The patient undergoes regular blood tests that determine the amount of each drug in her system and thus the daily dosages necessary to achieve therapeutic levels. Because "tight," or perfect, control of seizures with drugs can cause psychosis or an exaggeration of Geschwind's syndrome, the goal of anticonvulsant treatment is usually to reduce the frequency of seizures, not to stop them altogether. According to Edith Kaplan, "Many doctors think it's better for a patient to have a seizure now and then, rather than no seizures at all."

Doctors seek the combination of drugs that lessens each individual's TLE seizures with the fewest side effects. The most common drugs used for TLE today are Tegretol (carbamazepine), which was first marketed in the U.S. in 1974, Dilantin (phenytoin), available since 1938, and various forms of the barbiturate phenobarbital, available since 1912, all of which Charlie, Jill, and Gloria have tried. Charlie's doctor quickly settled on a modest dose of Tegretol, which Charlie has taken with good results for twelve years. During the first several years of Jill's TLE, she tried numerous anticonvulsants, alone and in combination, without finding any that worked well. Gloria, who has taken many anticonvulsants over decades, now takes Mysoline, a phenobarbital, and Dilantin. Too much or too little of any of these drugs can cause unpleasant side effects, and at high doses they are toxic, producing rapid involuntary eye movements, dizziness, clumsiness, tremor, dulling of intellect, forgetfulness, and stupor. Even in ordinary doses, Dilantin can cause excess growth of the gums, coarsening of facial features, thickening of body hair, skin rashes, and anemia; over many years it softens bones and alters lymph nodes. Possible side effects of Tegretol include allergies, double vision, gastrointestinal irritation, loss of bone marrow, reduced production of white blood cells, and liver damage. Phenobarbital can cause confusion, lethargy, and depression.

Because of the numerous side effects of existing anticonvulsants and the poor success rate of these drugs with TLE, research neurologists continually test new drugs on TLE patients who agree to participate in experimental studies, hoping for a miracle cure. Most of these studies are devoted to TLE because it is the form of epilepsy most difficult to treat. John Kuehnle, an expert in psychopharmacology, believes that discovery of "a magic bullet drug for TLE, something like lithium for manic-depressive illness, would really help in its diagnosis as well as its treatment." Some epilepsy drugs have been successful in treating other disorders; Tegretol, for instance, is prescribed for manic-depressive illness, mania (an affective disorder involving intense activity and hallucinations, often religious in tone, that alternates with depression in manic-depressive illness), and panic disorder. When these patients respond well to anticonvulsants, some doctors wonder whether they might actually have TLE.

Psychotherapy is often offered in combination with anticonvulsants because it is thought to help TLE patients adjust to living with their brain disorder. Charlie has never felt a need for psychotherapy, but both Gloria and Jill have undergone therapy for years. Once a week a van outfitted for the handicapped arrives at Gloria's house to drive her to the office of a psychiatrist. Like all of Gloria's doctors, he must make himself endlessly available to her on the phone. A year after Jill's diagnosis, she began having psychotherapy one to four times a month with Spiers, whom she met when Schomer, hoping to locate her seizure focus, sent her to him for a two-hour battery of neuropsychological tests. These tests, part of the workup done at Beth Israel Hospital on TLE patients being considered for epilepsy surgery, ascertain the functions of different brain regions. Tension built inside her as Spiers ran her through scores of questions about numbers, words, and pictures. "His testing strips you of everything," she recalled later. "Paul gets into all the different parts of your mind." When he finally said she could take a break, she began to weep. "I feel so frustrated and inadequate," she cried. "I can't do anything right anymore. I feel violated, like everybody in the world is just poking around in me." She and Spiers began talk therapy soon afterward.

The aim of her therapy, both agreed, was to enable her to distinguish her psychological problems from the depression, mood swings, and strange mental effects caused by her neurological disorder. Her neurological and psychological problems interact, so that it is difficult for her to tease the two apart. "Real emotional things and seizures and epilepsy get all washed up together, so it's hard to sort them out," she explained. Her reluctance to go out with men, for instance, could be a psychodynamic issue related to her fear of repeating her parents' unhappy marriage, or a result of fatigue due to multiple seizures, or a sign of interictal hyposexuality. In her case, according to Spiers, it is a combination of the three.

In therapy with Jill, Spiers took an unorthodox approach. He did not establish a regular appointment with her but encouraged her to call him whenever she felt the need. "When I feel lousy," she said, "I go to Paul's office. If I put my head on his desk, it means I feel really bad." After he left Beth Israel Hospital several years ago to become a research scientist at the Massachusetts Institute of Technology, he stopped charging her for therapy sessions, she said. He accepted free parking in her downtown corporate lot. They had lunch together occasionally. In dealing with her problems, he modeled himself on her mother, who, he believed, contributed to Jill's problems by "backing her into corners and telling her she wasn't good enough. With that background, Jill is understandably going to be reclusive, withdrawn, secretive, sensitive to rejection, and somewhat depressed."

Unlike the stereotypical passive therapist, Spiers was pushy and demanding with Jill. He dealt with her inability to save any money by making budgets for her and demanding that she arrange to have 7 percent of each paycheck automatically withdrawn and deposited into an inaccessible account. He pressured her to go on dates with new men, and he called her the morning after to see if she had followed through. "Jill needs to be backed into corners," he explained, "because she's used to keeping herself in a bind. When I want Jill to do something, I have to trap her, so she can't avoid making a decision. When it comes time to do something new in therapy, if I say, 'OK, this week we want you to go out and work on socializing more,' most people would go to the movies with one person, go to dinner with another, and go hang out in a nightclub. But with Jill, I have to say, 'OK, *this* is how we're gonna do it,' and help her set it up so it's inescapable. Her natural tendency is to retreat. I have to get her to make commitments to other people. If she puts money down to rent a house on the Cape for a week with a group, it's hard to back out: she loses a lot of money and disappoints others if she doesn't go."

Spiers has helped her through crises large and small. She called him on the one occasion, about five years after her diagnosis, when she was seriously considering suicide. She had been experiencing many seizures, losing sleep, and suffering from eye, neck, and head pain, chronic nausea, lethargy, and tremendous anxiety. She had trouble walking: at work, suddenly aware she was weaving, she had to concentrate simply on moving in a straight line. One morning, she awoke feeling that she could not rise from the bed. She saw visions of colors. She had no appetite. She could barely speak. "It was one of my black moods when I can't imagine getting to the next day," she recalled. "I wanted to take all my medicines at once. I really wanted to die." She dialed Spiers' office number and said, "I'm afraid this awful feeling won't go away. I can't go on like this. If I don't get better, I'm going to jump off my roof!"

"Don't jump off your roof," he shouted, as she recalls the conversation. He instructed her to go to a coffee shop near his office where, an hour later, they met and talked. On a napkin, he outlined a plan for the following year. She would try more anticonvulsants, in combination with several antidepressants, and she would be hospitalized for several weeks to have long-term EEG monitoring, part of the workup preparatory to the surgery for TLE. Relieved to have a plan to live by, Jill calmed down.

"I don't know what I would do without that man," Jill said later, her animated face radiating energy. "Paul has been the most help to me of anybody." Insofar as it affects her emotions, TLE may even underlie her unusually close, dependent relationship with the therapist, who himself said, "Jill is alone in the world—except for me."

If anticonvulsants fail to reduce the number or intensity of a patient's TLE seizures, some doctors try electroconvulsive therapy—ECT, or "shock treatment"—which helps a small proportion of patients with TLE. Other neurologists prescribe hormones. The exact relationship between hormone levels and TLE is not known, but some doctors suspect that seizures or seizure focuses affect the function of the hypothalamus, the temporolimbic structure that regulates hormones through the pituitary gland. Normal fluctuations of hormones in the body are known to influence seizure frequency, and seizures in turn affect the levels of hormones. According to doctors, 50 percent of women with TLE have irregular or no menstrual periods, and 50 percent of men with TLE have low levels of the male hormone testosterone; both effects hamper fertility. Many women with TLE also have ovarian cysts, which are believed to be caused by scars in the hypothalamus; Gloria and Jill have each had several such cysts removed. Pregnancy and birth control pills both affect seizure frequency in women. Mary Garth, the concert violinist whose TLE was not diagnosed for twenty years, said that the only times she consistently felt well during those decades were during her three pregnancies. She had no idea why, but her doctors now speculate that the hormone changes that occur in pregnancy acted as a natural anticonvulsant. In a few cases, people with abnormal hormone levels but no history of seizures of any kind have had their hormonal problem successfully treated with anticonvulsant drugs.

Further evidence of the link between seizures and hormones is catameneal epilepsy, in which a woman's seizures intensify or occur only prior to or during menstruation. Jill's TLE is catameneal. Before she developed the disorder, her menstrual periods never bothered her; now she has an increase in seizures before her period every other month. "I get wild, anxious, and unable to control my emotions," she said. "I have a headache for three days. I can't sleep well: I wake up ten or twelve times a night." Hoping to treat this problem, Schomer referred her to an endocrinologist, who tested her and found a physical basis for this mental change: the level of the female hormone progesterone in her system lowers abnormally for unknown reasons six days before menstruation, causing her seizures to intensify until her period comes. Then, abruptly, she is free of seizures and feels euphoric for a day or two. Hoping to reduce her premenstrual seizures by changing the way her seizures and hormone levels interact, the endocrinologist prescribed a fertility drug, to no avail. Next he tried giving her progesterone pills for the six days before her period. For several months, the hormone reduced the number of days per month that she felt badly from ten to one. But this effect soon wore off, as her system gradually accommodated itself to the hormone infusions. The progesterone also had the side effect of making her lethargic, so the doctor advised her to stop taking it. Jill, who had been reluctant to take artificial hormones, was relieved.

Should all other available treatments fail to help a TLE patient, doctors may consider surgery. Epilepsy surgery has a long history: from the late Stone Age until the early twentieth century, physicians performed trepanning, or trepanation, which involved boring holes in an epileptic's skull in a vain and life-threatening attempt to free the demons that were thought to cause seizures. The brain operation used for TLE today is similar to that performed in the 1930s by Penfield in Montreal. At a number of major medical centers around the world, neurosurgeons use a scalpel and a suction device to remove the brain area that contains the seizure focus, a mass of tissue often as large as a fist, in an attempt to reduce or end seizures. Because the abnormal activity generated by an epileptic scar can damage surrounding tissue, many doctors aim to take out as much tissue as possible without affecting a patient's essential functions. Consequently, neurosurgeons often remove most of an entire brain lobe in one hemisphere, usually the temporal lobe, which is the region most likely to develop a seizure focus; less frequently, all or part of one frontal, occipital, or parietal lobe is removed. For most other surgical procedures the patient is given general anesthesia, but because of the need for getting accurate EEG readings and mapping brain functions during this procedure, the patient, though sedated, is conscious throughout.

Only a small minority of TLE patients are considered for this operation, which has been performed, in conjunction with the EEG, on fewer than six thousand patients since 1939. The success rate has been consistent: slightly more than a third of survivors become seizure-free and are able to go off anticonvulsants; another third of patients have significantly fewer seizures while remaining on drugs; and slightly less than a third stay the same as before or worsen. Worsening usually means more frequent seizures and the introduction of new kinds of seizures; in rare cases it involves lasting difficulties with thinking and remembering. An exceptionally low number of patients who have the operation—far fewer than 1 percent—die as a result, largely because it does not involve general anesthesia, which is a frequent cause of surgical death.

The lobectomy itself takes six to eight hours, and the preparation (the "surgical workup") and recovery take between one and five years. The workup involves numerous brain tests to determine the location of the major arteries, veins, and language areas, all of which the neurosurgeon must avoid. Patients also undergo intensive long-term EEG monitoring, sometimes with attached video machines, which enable doctors to correlate a patient's EEG recording with his clinical seizure state. Recent technological advances have enabled some patients to take EEG machines home. In a process called telemetry, electrodes are glued to the scalp, the head is bandaged, and the patient is given a portable, battery-operated pack, worn over the shoulder, that takes EEG readings for days. If doctors are still unable to determine the hemisphere in which seizures start, surgeons may insert "strip electrodes" through burr holes drilled in the skull or may surgically implant "depth electrodes" inside the brain, both of which techniques can afford more precise EEG readings. Near the end of the workup, surgeons often stimulate the brain with low currents of electricity in an attempt to locate epileptic tissue more accurately by replicating seizures. To be considered for the operation, patients must meet strict criteria: their seizures must be sufficiently incapacitating to justify the time, cost, and risks of surgery; and their seizure focuses must be in only one hemisphere and distinct from essential brain areas. Since bilateral removal of any lobe would cause dramatic and disabling functional losses, only unilateral lobectomies are performed.

Several hundred of these operations for TLE are performed each year in the United States. Doctors disagree as to the procedure's value. In the early 1960s Geschwind reported, "Over all the years that I have been interested in TLE, I have seen only a handful of patients for whom I would consider surgery," and in each case "it has been a difficult decision." Today, doctors who have few surgical patients, such as those outside major medical centers, tend to be suspicious of epilepsy surgery. Edwards considers the operation dangerous and often unnecessary. "The whole temporal lobectomy business is way overdone," he said. "I've seen a lot of *post*temporal lobectomy patients, and those from hospitals in Boston or Hanover have all come back worse, with neurological deficits such as language or memory problems. One woman has had two or three temporal lobectomies; they kept picking out more brain tissue each time. I even saw one of Penfield's former patients, who had been a real estate agent. Penfield took out too much of his left temporal lobe, so he now has so much aphasia [loss of language] that he can function only as a janitor." The man's seizures remain the same as before the operation. "He's very angry, because his operation was done in the 1960s, just before Tegretol came out, and his seizures are now controllable with Tegretol. The surgery is better today than it was then, but still, if you just wait another year or two, we're going to have better medicines. I don't see why you should lose part of your brain unless the seizure disorder is completely disabling." Edwards refers the small percentage of his patients whose seizures are not controllable by other means to Yale–New Haven Hospital to be worked up for the surgery. He chose this hospital because its "doctors are much more conservative" in screening patients for the operation than are doctors at other nearby epilepsy centers. So far, none of his patients has been accepted for TLE surgery. "The doctors have always said, 'We can't operate because this isn't a good candidate,' and that's just fine with me."

On the other hand, many doctors at medical centers where temporal lobectomies are performed consider the procedure underutilized. At Beth Israel Hospital, for instance, Jill has been encouraged to have the surgical workup, and the neurosurgeon Howard Blume, who performs about twenty temporal lobectomies for epilepsy each year, estimates that a hundred thousand people with TLE in the United States alone could benefit from a temporal lobectomy. According to Blume's colleague Schomer, "Many more people could be helped by this procedure." George Ojemann, a neurosurgeon at the University of Washington in Seattle, estimates that fewer than 2 percent of potential candidates undergo epilepsy surgery. In many cases, according to Allen Wyler, a Tennessee neurosurgeon, "the risks of surgery are less than the risks of continued seizures."

Like anticonvulsant drugs, epilepsy surgery is intended to relieve seizures, not the traits of Geschwind's syndrome. And in most cases, according to doctors, neither treatment does have much effect on personality. But there are exceptions. As Kaplan pointed out, perfect drug control occasionally enhances the traits, for unknown reasons, and successful surgery sometimes reduces the traits, perhaps because the scar causing them has been removed. A common long-term effect of the operation is improved overall neurological functioning, which is thought to occur because epileptic tissue interferes with normal brain function. An eighteen-year-old woman who had a temporal lobectomy at Beth Israel Hospital soon afterward experienced a general leavening of mood and outlook. Not only did her IQ rise, but she developed an interest in sex, and her aggression and hyperreligiosity were muted. Before the surgery she was "dour, nasty, and grudge-holding," according to Spiers, "and now I can't wipe the smile off her face." Such exceptions usually involve young patients with relatively recent onset of epilepsy, which suggests that the traits solidify only after longtime epileptic activity. Because the surgery tends to produce better results in younger patients with newer seizure disorders, and because long-term seizures can bring on a deepening of Geschwind's syndrome and a schizophreniform psychosis, neurosurgeons prefer to operate on people with TLE as soon as possible. According to Kuehnle, an early temporal lobectomy preempts the development of Geschwind's syndrome. In older patients who have had successful surgery, the traits often persist, probably because, in Bear's view, while the scar that underlies the seizures is gone, the

altered neuronal circuits that govern the personality changes
remain. In any case, personality changes after treatment are
incidental, according to neurosurgeons, whose explicit goal in
surgery is always to end the disorder's symptoms—seizures—
never to alter the associated traits.

In the 1960s, however, a neurosurgeon proposed a different
kind of TLE surgery. The main goal of this operation was to
alter personality. The procedure, which involved burning out a
small temporolimbic region involved in rage and sexuality in
both cerebral hemispheres of people with TLE, was not neurosurgery, but psychosurgery. Psychosurgery began, as did neurosurgery, in the late nineteenth century, when the discovery of
anesthesia and improved cleanliness made surgical procedures
reasonably safe. But the two kinds of surgery differ in their
aims: neurosurgery involves surgical treatments for disorders
of the nervous system, which consists of the brain and spine,
while psychosurgery involves surgical treatments for disorders
of the psyche, or mind. In psychosurgery, a surgeon attempts to
remove certain traits, such as extreme aggression or sexuality,
by altering or removing brain regions that, on the basis of animal studies, have been shown to contribute to these traits—literally changing the patient's mind. The same procedure could
in fact be viewed as either neurosurgery or psychosurgery,
depending on whether its goal is to treat an illness or to "treat"
personality.

Unfortunately for psychosurgeons, personality is not as
amenable to surgical repair as is bodily tissue. The best known
psychosurgical procedure, the prefrontal leucotomy, popularly
known in the United States as a "lobotomy," is a case in point.
Introduced as a treatment for schizophrenia in 1935 by Egas
Moniz, a Portugese doctor, the lobotomy involved scrambling
the frontal lobes of a conscious patient with a picklike knife
inserted through the forehead. Moniz, who was a neurologist,
not a surgeon, did not carry out the procedure himself but
instead supervised a young surgeon, Almeida Lima. Moniz
soon reported that the operation made agitated patients calm.
As a result of his optimistic report, this procedure or something like it was soon performed in many other countries in
Europe, Asia, and South America, as well as in the United
States.

In the spring of 1936, in Washington, D.C., while reading a French medical journal, Walter Freeman, an American neuropathologist, came upon Moniz's first article describing the new procedure. Freeman showed the article to a colleague, James Winston Watts, a neurosurgeon at George Washington University Hospital, and the two men decided to try Moniz's procedure as soon as possible. Freeman wrote to Moniz telling him of their intention. The American then ordered from a medical-instrument maker in Paris several of the surgical knives that Moniz had designed, which were called *leucotomes*, from the Greek for "white matter" and "knife." In September, Freeman and Watts jointly operated on their first patient, a sixty-three-year-old woman from Kansas who had been diagnosed as agitated and depressed. Within three weeks of the procedure, they reported that the lobotomy had ended her anxiety and fear. Although she had also lost her ability to speak coherently, Freeman pronounced her "cured."

Encouraged by what they considered their initial success, Freeman and Watts soon carried out the same procedure on five more agitated patients. These patients all became less worried, more placid, and easier to care for, the doctors reported. While conceding that they were not certain if these patients could still "function satisfactorily" in society, the doctors went on to perform one thousand more such operations.

Freeman's new operation was soon widely considered a beneficial treatment for schizophrenia and lauded as a possible "cure" for robbery and criminal violence. The neuropathologist was gifted at self-promotion, and magazines and major newspapers across the country published positive stories about him. The procedure quickly grew in popularity. While fewer than three hundred lobotomies were performed in the United States by 1942, more than ten thousand were performed by 1949, and nearly double that number by 1951. The number of lobotomies reached its peak in the years 1949 to 1952, when roughly five thousand such operations were performed annually on mentally ill people. In 1949, when the seventy-five-year-old Moniz was awarded the Nobel Prize for Physiology or Medicine for initiating the prefrontal leucotomy, the procedure still seemed like a medical breakthrough. Although some prominent American surgeons and psychiatrists privately considered the procedure bar-

baric and lacking in medical justification, practically no negative information was published about it in the United States during the first ten years.

However, as the glow wore off, doctors and the public began to realize that lobotomy succeeded by overkill. It not only calmed patients but also left them incapable of doing much of anything, even the simplest of tasks. As Freeman and Watts admitted, "Every patient probably loses something by this operation, some spontaneity, some sparkle, some flavor of the personality." After lobotomy, the doctors noted, a patient cannot give "advice on any important matter. . . . There is something childlike in [his] directness and ingenuousness. . . . [He is] practical and uninspired." While memory, which relies on the temporal lobes, was usually unaffected by this frontal-lobe operation, many unpleasant changes occurred: patients became restless, apathetic, inattentive, distractible, emotionally volatile, uninhibited, and unable to think or plan as they had before. Some patients died. Others, who at first seemed to improve, suffered "relapses" several months after the operation and had to be operated on a second and even third time. Many patients remained institutionalized. Of those who could go home, most were unable to work and required nursing care. Some patients developed seizures, probably because brain tissue had been damaged by the surgeon's instrument.

Patients' reactions to the operation were hardly without precedent, in both animal experimentation and human experience. As early as the 1880s, Hughlings Jackson's colleague Sir David Ferrier had described monkeys and apes whose frontal lobes had been surgically removed as "apathetic or dull, or doz[ing] off to sleep, responding only to the sensations or impressions of the moment . . . [making] purposeless wanderings to and fro." People who lost all or part of both frontal lobes accidentally or, like Penfield's sister, in surgery for a brain tumor underwent similar changes, becoming disoriented, distractible, and unable to plan.

Still, Freeman denied the limitations of the operation he had promoted so enthusiastically. By 1953, although he had abandoned the use of prefrontal lobotomy on longtime schizophrenic patients or on schizophrenics who hallucinated, he continued to perform lobotomies on less impaired patients. In search of other surgical treatments for the mentally ill, he tried an amygdalectomy, which involved removing the amygdala, a temporal-lobe structure involved in emotions. But this procedure did not help chronic schizophrenics either. Next, speculating that the region *between* the temporal and frontal lobes was at the root of schizophrenia, he tried destroying fibers there, to no avail. Freeman performed his last operation in 1967, in California, at age seventy-two. The patient was a woman on whom he had done lobotomies twice before, in 1946 and 1956. At the start of her third lobotomy, Freeman's surgical instrument ripped a major blood vessel in her brain, causing an internal hemorrhage. Hours later, the woman died, and Freeman's surgical privileges were revoked.

Psychosurgery began its fall from favor during the 1950s, not only because of the incapacitating effects of Moniz's operation, but also because of the introduction of drugs that reduced some of the effects of schizophrenia, starting with Thorazine, which was developed in 1954. By the mid-1960s, most forms of psychosurgery were in disrepute.

Yet Vernon Mark, a neurosurgeon then in his early forties who with positions at Harvard Medical School and several Boston hospitals seemed on his way to the top of his field, wished to attempt a new kind of psychosurgery on people with TLE. Instead of removing the symptoms of schizophrenia, as Freeman had hoped, Mark intended to remove what he considered a symptom of TLE, violent rage. He planned to do this by destroying parts of a temporolimbic structure that Freeman had removed in schizophrenics, the amygdala, which modulates emotions. The amygdala, whose name comes from the Greek for "almond" because of its size and shape, is located in duplicate—one amygdala in each hemisphere—in the front of the limbic system. When the amygdala of a monkey or a cat is stimulated with a probe, the animal usually attacks whatever is nearby, whether a stuffed animal or a man. Similarly, electrical stimulation of the human amygdala in surgery produces powerful emotions—usually rage, sometimes fear or sexual arousal. In 1961 a patient reported during amygdala stimulation, "I don't know what came over me. I felt like an animal." Another patient cried angrily, "I feel like I want to get up from this chair! I want to hit something. I want to get something and just tear it up. Take it so

I won't!" To prevent herself from shredding her scarf, the patient handed it to a doctor. In return he gave her a pile of papers, which she ripped to pieces. "I don't like to feel like this!" she shouted. When the doctor reduced the current in the electrode to her brain, the patient suddenly smiled.

"Feel better?" the doctor asked.

"A little bit," the patient replied.

"How were you feeling a moment ago?"

"I wanted to get up and run. I wanted to hit something, tear up something, anything. I had no control of myself."

Literally controlling her mind, the doctor again raised the current to her amygdala. "Don't let me hit you!" she pleaded. "Quit holding me! I'm getting up! You'd better get somebody else if you want to hold me!" She raised her arm, as if to strike him. "I'm going to hit you!" The doctor again reduced the current, and the woman said apologetically, "I couldn't help it. I wanted to slap your face. I don't like to be done like that."

Mark's plan was to gather a group of patients with both TLE and histories of violent behavior and to perform on each of them an experimental psychosurgical procedure that he called a "bilateral amygdala destruction," or amygdalotomy, in hopes of ending their seizures and reducing their aggression. The foundation for this operation was the evidence of personality changes in laboratory animals after removal of both amygdalas, an operation called a bilateral amygdalectomy. Following this operation, rhesus monkeys undergo a major emotional change. They lose all aggression and become extremely docile, uninterested in fighting even when attacked. Apparently losing short-term memory for the things they see and eat, they become visually indiscriminate, inspecting everything over and over, and highly oral, stuffing anything possible into their mouths. Sexually they become insatiable, mounting whatever is in their paths, including metal, their own feces, and hissing snakes. These changes, which are known collectively as the Klüver-Bucy syndrome, after the two scientists who described them in 1939, have occurred time and time again in monkeys after bilateral amygdalectomies.

To Norman Geschwind, the Klüver-Bucy syndrome suggested that the region around the amygdala is a crucial connection point between sensations, instincts, and emotions,

where decisions are made, for instance, about whether to flee
or to fight. Changes similar to the Klüver-Bucy syndrome are
seen in other animals following the same procedure: some rats
no longer kill mice; mallard ducks lose their fear of humans;
and cats copulate with chickens. Researchers, noting that the
reduced aggression and increased sexuality of the Klüver-Bucy
syndrome are mirror images of features of Geschwind's syndrome, speculate that overstimulation of the amygdala by
epileptic activity creates an excess of connections between
senses and instincts, contributing to the TLE traits. According
to Bear, "TLE, frequently a condition in which amygdalar neurons have acquired a lowered threshold for discharge, is in a
general sense the converse of removing or destroying the
amygdala."

Mark believed that destruction of the amygdala would
reverse the traits of Geschwind's syndrome, but he, like his fore-
runners Moniz and Freeman, was selective in his reading of
past experiments. While he noted that monkeys became less
aggressive after amygdalectomies, he did not address how the
other changes in monkeys—such as oral and sexual cravings—
would play themselves out in humans. He dismissed the rele-
vance of other animal studies, such as those showing that bilateral destruction of the amygdala in cats makes them more—not
less—savage and aggressive. Mark also seemed to disregard
some human studies. In the few cases in which both temporal
lobes, including both amygdalas, had been removed from
humans, a human version of the Klüver-Bucy syndrome
resulted: patients became profoundly apathetic, and their memories were severely impaired. The most celebrated case
occurred in New Haven in 1953. A patient known as "H.M.,"
whose surgeon removed both temporal lobes in an attempt to
lessen his disabling epilepsy, suffered a complete and incapacitating loss of his ability to form new memories. Previously an
electrician's assistant, H.M. was now unable to perform even
simple tasks.

Mark viewed the possibility of bilateral amygdalotomies on
violent TLE patients with great optimism, predicting that the
procedure would enable society to address its broader problem
of violence. In a statement published in the *Journal of the American Medical Association* in 1967, he and two colleagues from

Harvard Medical School, William Sweet, another neurosurgeon, and Frank Ervin, a neuropsychiatrist, speculated that brain damage had caused the urban riots that erupted across the country the previous summer. The doctors suggested testing and studying individual rioters "to pinpoint, diagnose," and "treat" with psychosurgery "people with low violence thresholds before they contribute to further tragedies." This was an "unfortunate statement," according to Bear, "because it swept under the rug the real issues, culture and poverty, and it raised the specter of burning out parts of these people's brains."

Three years later, Mark and Ervin published *Violence and the Brain*, a controversial book that took "a biologically-oriented approach to the problem of human violence," describing violence as a medical problem and a symptom, and calling a bilateral amygdalotomy an experimental treatment for violence. According to the authors, "an appreciable percentage of the relatively few individuals guilty of repeated personal violence are to be found in [the] 5 to 10 percent of the population whose brains do not function in a perfectly normal way." After studying the records of several hundred violent prisoners and psychiatric inpatients, the doctors concluded that violent people have "damaged or malfunctioning brains." Mark and Ervin called the tendency toward impulsive violence an "episodic dyscontrol syndrome," which they viewed as similar to TLE because of the association of that disorder with increased aggression. The episodic dyscontrol syndrome consisted of four traits—a history of physical assaults, such as beating wives or children; alcohol abuse; impulsive sexual behavior; and auto accidents and moving violations—and was caused, they theorized, by abnormalities in the limbic system. Speculating that "the production of small focal areas of destruction" in the temporolimbic brain would "eliminate dangerous behavior in assaultive or violent patients," the doctors wrote that they hoped ultimately to solve "the most threatening problem in our world today" by "controlling" violence with medical means.

To this end, in the mid-1960s Mark had established the Neuro-Research Foundation, its goal being "the diagnosis and treatment of persons with poor control of violent impulses," and had sought federal money for research into the relationship between violence and abnormal electrical activity in the brain.

In the late 1960s, when he applied to the National Institute of Mental Health for several hundred thousand dollars with which to experiment on humans with brain disorders and tendencies toward violence, the NIMH initially turned him down. His Harvard colleague William Sweet then took the request directly to the federal government, lobbying Elliot Richardson, President Nixon's Secretary of Health, Education and Welfare, for financial support. Richardson, who was a neighbor of Mark's, approved $500,000 for Mark's research in the 1970 HEW budget, and persuaded the NIMH to reverse its decision. Between 1970 and 1972, the NIMH granted Mark and Sweet nearly one million dollars for violence research. Nearly two hundred thousand dollars in additional research funding came in 1971 from the Law Enforcement Assistance Administration, the branch of the Justice Department responsible for prisons. Technically, the funds were awarded as "contracts" rather than "grants," thus avoiding the problem of peer review.

Even before receiving most of this federal money, Mark had begun his experiment in "treating" violence. Starting in 1965, he carried out bilateral amygdalotomies on at least eight people, all inpatients at one time or another on a locked ward at Massachusetts General Hospital, where he had accumulated patients with abnormal brain activity and a history of violence. In December 1969, Gloria became a patient on that ward.

Then thirty-nine years old, Gloria had been a candidate for a bilateral amygdalotomy since 1967, the year her surgical workup began. That spring, Mark had sent her for a series of brain scans in order to determine the location of her seizure activity, brain structures, arteries, and veins, preparatory to surgery. He considered her a good candidate for the experimental procedure because of her history of "sexual excesses" and "assaultiveness," contributing to the diagnosis of "episodic dyscontrol syndrome" as well as her seizures and abnormal EEG. In 1967 she had consented to one brain scan but, fearful of the idea of brain surgery, refused to allow technicians to carry out the remaining ones. Two and a half years later, she was admitted to the hospital for depression and suicidal feelings. Although she was still afraid of having her brain stimulated or burned, this time she was far less inclined to refuse the operation Mark had proposed.

One reason she agreed to the surgery, she said years later,

was that she had no idea that it was experimental. In fact, she believed that it was a proven treatment for TLE. In this regard, she was typical of Mark's amygdalotomy patients, according to the neuropsychologist Stephan Chorover, a professor at Massachusetts Institute of Technology and a critic of psychosurgery. "Gloria and the other patients Mark operated on saw themselves as patients of a doctor," Chorover said, "but the doctor's view was much more complicated; to him, Gloria was both a patient *and* an experimental subject."

Moreover, Gloria did not have the benefit of today's stringent rules regarding a patient's "informed consent," rules that were instated in part because of the results of the psychosurgery that Mark performed. In the 1960s, explicit consent procedures did not exist; for instance, it was not necessary then, as it is now, to have a patient's written consent before a surgical procedure could be performed. According to Gloria's medical records, Mark did not seek her written permission for the operation. He did, however, discuss with her the risks and the probability of success. "I have spoken to the patient about the risks including infection, neurological brain deficit, memory loss and even death," he wrote on the day the operation began. "She understands the limitations and expectations of surgery—about 70 percent chance of some improvement—and is willing to undergo the risks of surgery for the possible benefits." In fact, since Mark's procedure was experimental, it is unlikely that any figure existed as to its potential for success. The figure he used, 70 percent, was the rate of success for the standard temporal lobectomy; decade after decade in hospital after hospital, roughly two-thirds of patients who had that unilateral procedure showed at least mild improvement. Temporal lobectomy, however, was not the procedure that Mark was about to perform.

Mark's pioneering procedure involved several stages and took place over several months. First, in an operation involving general anesthesia, he implanted multiple electrodes in the patient's brain. He left electrodes in the brain far longer than anyone had done before, for weeks or even months. Once the patient had recovered from the surgery, Mark used the implanted electrodes to stimulate the conscious patient's brain, sending mild electric currents down them repeatedly for days or

weeks, observing and recording the results. This part of the procedure was both diagnostic and experimental: Mark wanted to
know specifically which areas would, when stimulated, produce
reactions similar to the patient's usual seizures, and he was also
curious about how multiple stimulations affect the emotional
brain.

In the course of stimulating his patients' brains, Mark
elicited abrupt attacks of rage, sexual feeling, and fear similar to
those elicited by earlier doctors. He also discovered that he could
stop the violent behavior he had initiated simply by stimulating
certain parts of the amygdala and hippocampus, a nearby, sea-
horse-shaped structure involved in learning, memory, and hormones. In carrying out these stimulations, Chorover later
explained, Mark was in "an unparalleled situation. First, he had
human subjects with electrodes in their brains. Second, he had
an incredible interest in the effects of brain stimulation and
brain lesions on personality, mood, and behavior, especially such
emotionally laden activities as violence and sexuality. Third, he
believed—he couldn't have known better at the time, although
everybody knows better now—that you could stimulate the brain
at low levels with impunity." Mark did not realize that repeatedly
stimulating the brain can in fact create epileptic scars; this "kindling" effect was not discovered until 1973.

After several weeks or months of these stimulations, Mark
carried out the actual amygdala destruction, first in one hemisphere, then in the other. Each amygdalotomy was done under
local anesthetic and took place over several days. This part of the
procedure involved sending several currents of heat through the
implanted electrode that rested in the patient's amygdala,
destroying tissue there. To Mark, burning tissue seemed preferable to cutting and removing it, as in a lobectomy, which is far
more invasive and involves far more brain tissue. Finally, the
patient again went under general anesthesia and the surgeon
removed the implanted electrodes.

Gloria's procedure began at Massachusetts General Hospital
on December 2, 1969. Early that morning, Mark, a tall man with
dark, thinning hair, scrubbed and donned his surgical garb and
entered the surgical theater where Gloria lay, unconscious, on
her left side, facing an anesthesiologist. Over the right side of her
head, the neurosurgeon sliced her shaven scalp, drew the skin

back, and secured it with clips. He drilled several holes in her skull over the area of her amygdala. Through each hole he inserted a hollow needle that contained a thin, flexible electrode strand with several metal nubs near its tip, each of which would convey electrical information from—and deliver currents of electricity and heat to—a tiny part of her brain. When the needle approached what he believed was her right amygdala, he withdrew it, leaving the electrode strand deep inside her brain.

To locate her amygdala, which was equivalent to finding a grain of rice in a bowl of rice pudding without disturbing the pudding, Mark had used a technique for charting brain structures called *stereotaxy*, from the Greek for "ordering three-dimensional space." Prior to the implantation he pinned to her head a metal scaffolding called a stereotactic machine. He then injected a dye into her brain and took X rays of her temporolimbic region with a camera attached to the machine. Using the ruled marks along the ribs of the machine as a measure, he located the amygdala and other brain structures visible on the X ray. This charting technique was first used by Jackson's English colleague Sir Victor Horsley in experiments on animals in the early twentieth century; its use on humans dates from the 1940s. For diagnostic purposes stereotaxy is generally not harmful, but when used surgically, Bear commented two decades after Gloria's operation, it had a "fundamental flaw." The stereotactic machine "just wasn't that great. If you stick an electrode in the brain, a three-dimensional structure, the probability that you're going to hit the epileptic focus square on is very low. Even if you hit the amygdala, it might not be the right part. The electrode usually didn't go through the heart of the epileptic focus, so that the heat lesions Mark made destroyed fibers and nerve cells and changed the neuronal path of the person's typical seizure, but they didn't change the ultimate outcome." In short, patients continued to seize.

Following the first electrode implantation, Mark cleaned Gloria's head wound, closed her scalp, removed the stereotactic machine, and placed her head in a sterile headrest. In contrast to the EEG taken a day before with ordinary surface electrodes, which was normal, an EEG reading from the implanted electrodes showed several areas of abnormal electrical activity, indicating that her epileptic activity was deep in her brain.

Like most patients in whom Mark implanted electrodes, Gloria experienced initial pain and problems with memory, vision, and walking, all of which soon went away. By December 5 Gloria had returned to normal, according to Mark's notes, and she "roused up quickly" in protest when he mentioned the possibility of doing a lumbar puncture, a painful spinal examination that she had undergone before and refused to have again.

During the week of December 12, the neurosurgeon stimulated her amygdalar region every day. He sent repeated currents of mild electricity down the implanted electrodes and kept a notebook of what happened to Gloria and to her EEG. According to a doctor who saw Gloria in 1971 and who had access to her records, "Much data was obtained from the[sc] studies." Mark elicited numerous seizures typical of those she had experienced for years, consisting of bad smells, staring, hand-rubbing, grasping the medical staff near her bed, alterations in consciousness, and subsequent amnesia for the time of the seizure. He also induced numerous attacks of sudden aggressive or sexual feelings, which were not typical of Gloria's seizures, and which would in fact occur in anyone whose amygdala was stimulated with sufficient current in the right place. During a lengthy stimulation session on December 17, for instance, Gloria had a "violent episode." According to her chart, as Mark sent another electrical current toward her amygdala, she reached up and "grabbed the investigator violently." Gloria later recalled that she had felt sexually aroused and reached for a young male technician who was standing nearby. "I wanted to have [sexual] relations with him so bad," she said. "They had stimulated me a lot, stirred me up, and made me very passionate."

Later that day, she continued to have many brief seizural staring spells and became a problem on the ward. In the evening, she brandished a broken glass and threatened a nurse and a doctor. The doctor was able to calm her down and convinced her to go to sleep.

The next day, Mark transferred Gloria from the private Massachusetts General Hospital to Boston City Hospital, a public hospital in a poor neighborhood, where he was also on staff. "Mark shipped his patients to BCH if they became disruptive," Kuehnle said. Gloria considered the transfer a kind of punishment. A week earlier, after overhearing Massachusetts General staff discuss the possibility of moving her, she had told a social worker that she feared being "tricked into" going to Boston City Hospital. "She will use every power she has not to go," the social worker noted. "She feels she has been good here and should not be punished by a transfer right after surgery—that this will adversely affect her will to get better in the future. She feels that any machine at BCH could be brought here." The day the transfer occurred, this social worker noted the connection between the transfer and the "episode of violence," and she wrote in Gloria's chart, "It is unfortunate that patient's belief that transfer to BCH would be a punishment was so correct."

At the city hospital, Mark began the actual amygdalotomy, starting with her right hemisphere. On three separate days— December 20, 27, and 29—Mark made "destructive lesions," sending currents of heat between 150 and 170 degrees Fahrenheit to the tip of an implanted electrode for three to five minutes. During the creation of the first lesion, according to Mark, Gloria had a seizural starting spell, "an angry look," and she "thrashed about with her legs," perhaps because of the disturbance of brain activity produced by the heat. Between the creation of the first and second lesions, she slept nearly around the clock, seemed to have lost track of time, and continued to seize frequently. Her right leg moved "powerfully" during the second lesion, Mark noted, perhaps as a left-brain response to the burst of heat in her right hemisphere. After making the third lesion, Mark noted "EEG evidence of injury" but "no appreciative clinical change."

Her right amygdalotomy now done, Gloria was transferred from neurosurgery to psychiatry for her recovery from the trauma of brain surgery. During the first few weeks she had to relearn how to talk and, because her left leg was weak, how to walk. During this time, she continued to take the anticonvulsants Dilantin and Mysoline and the antipsychotic Stelazine. For unknown reasons, the electrodes remained in her right hemisphere for five more weeks, until February 4, 1970, when Mark removed them.

By the time she went home, in the spring of 1970, it was clear to everyone that the operation had hardly affected her, if it had affected her at all. Gloria was still Gloria. She continued to have many seizures daily. She remained angry—at her family, at her doctors, at strangers. Her personality had not changed. The reason, Bear said later, was that Mark had thus far operated on only her right hemisphere, the nondominant side of her brain, where large removals can occur without impairment of or alteration in function.

According to hospital records, Mark's colleagues encouraged Gloria to continue the procedure, to have her left amygdala destroyed. In November 1970, a doctor who saw her as an outpatient at the city hospital wrote in her chart, "At present she is contemplating [further] neurosurgery but has anxiety over whether operation might leave her crippled or whether it would be of benefit. She feels that she cannot trust her doctors although the essential risks and dangers have been well presented to her. She probably will not consent either to hospitalization or to surgery at present." Six weeks later, a psychiatrist noted that she "is depressed, anxious about repeat operation but hopefully, if this will have chance of help it can be done with aid of psychiatry service to help convince her of need for surgery. Refer to neurosurgery." In 1971, another doctor described her as being "incapacitated" by as many as one hundred seizures a day, and he recommended "electrolytic lesions to left amygdala."

Although these doctors apparently pressured her to continue the bilateral amygdalotomy, another doctor offered different advice. Sometime in 1971, Gloria recalled later, Kuehnle, who practiced psychiatry at the Harvard-affiliated McLean Hospital, "told me not to let Dr. Mark do the other side of my brain. Dr. Kuehnle said to me, 'You'll be *finished* if he touches your other side.' I said, 'Thanks for telling me.'" Kuehnle explained later that he had been taught that "you shouldn't do removals on both sides of the brain. But I had been wondering about Gloria's case, so at grand rounds one day I asked Geschwind, 'If the amygdalotomy doesn't work on one side, why shouldn't you do both?' He said, 'It shouldn't be done bilaterally; it affects people severely, altering appetites.'" Kuehnle's counsel gave Gloria the confidence to refuse the other half of the operation, in a real sense saving her mind.

For several more years, she said, Mark continued to encourage her to have the rest of the operation. In 1976, when she was admitted to Massachusetts General because of a broken leg, Mark visited her in her room. According to her recollection, he

said, "Gloria, as you know, your brain is still extensively damaged. Let me do your other side."

"No," she replied, fearing that the left amygdalotomy would
permanently damage her memory or thinking. "I told him to get
the hell out of my room. He wasn't even my doctor then: I was in
orthopedics, for my leg."

But two decades after the operation, Mark indicated that he
could not have encouraged her to continue it, because he had
decided at some point during the ten days of her right amygdalotomy that her problem was more complicated than TLE. "I didn't
complete the bilateral procedure on her because it was obvious
then that she's a sociopath, and we don't have any operation for
that." The term *sociopath*, which doctors have now abandoned in
favor of *antisocial personality disorder*, describes a person who
commits antisocial acts such as theft, assault, and promiscuity,
and who is then callous and indifferent, feeling neither guilt nor
fear of punishment. Mark based his new diagnosis on Gloria's
"spectacular" history of extreme anger and sexual activity.
Although she never actually killed anyone, "she would lie, steal,
cheat, murder, etcetera, and I'm being nice about it," he said. "In
thirty years [of practice] there are only two violent patients I want
to have *nothing* to do with, and she's one of them." Although his
colleagues had pressed her to have the left amygdalotomy as late
as 1971, Mark said that by late December 1969 he had viewed
Gloria's TLE, frontal-lobe damage, and "sociopathy" as "a devas-
tating concatenation of problems that is pretty much beyond the
pale of medicine." He added, however, that "Gloria is *not* insane.
If she were, we couldn't execute any killers, because they could all
plead not guilty by reason of insanity."

Nevertheless, in 1974 Gloria was sent to a hospital for the
criminally insane. Although this was not then the customary
treatment for diagnosed TLE patients, it had historical prece-
dents: into the nineteenth century, epileptics were frequently
confined in hospitals for the insane. Increasingly difficult to
manage, according to Mark, Gloria was committed in September 1974 to Bridgewater State Hospital for the Criminally
Insane, a maximum-security hospital and penitentiary in Massachusetts where the documentary *Titicut Follies* had been
filmed eight years earlier. The prison is legally for men only, but
a spokesperson for the Massachusetts penal department

acknowledged in 1988 that "because of overcrowding" several women were sent to Bridgewater in the early 1970s. Gloria, who knows the hospital's reputation for housing some of the state's most violent criminals, is ashamed that she was there, and she shushes anyone who brings it up in public.

The three months Gloria spent at Bridgewater were among the worst of her life. "I had a horrible-looking room," she said. "There was so little to eat I went down to ninety pounds." The rheumatoid arthritis that she had recently developed worsened dramatically due to the prison's dampness and cold. The circumstances of her release at Christmastime are not clear. "My father brought a lawyer to get me out," she recalled. Upon her release, she was moved to the Lemuel Shattuck Hospital, a state psychiatric facility that accepted women patients.

As the years wore on, Mark sought to reduce contact with her and gradually withdrew from her care. In the late 1970s, he referred her to his young colleague David Bear. The first day Bear met Gloria, her personality amazed him as an unbelievable exaggeration of Geschwind's syndrome. Bear considered her a clear case of TLE with possible frontal-lobe damage, and he disputed Mark's diagnosis of sociopathy. To Bear, Gloria is the opposite of a sociopath: rather than lacking feeling, she has deeper emotions than most people. "Gloria has performed anti-social acts," he said, "but she's *not* a sociopath. So-called sociopaths are lighthearted, never guilty or remorseful. She's so moral and religious" in her commitment to civic activism and spiritual meditation "that she *can't* be a sociopath." Unlike the "classic" sociopath, who appears normal, even attractive, at first but proves heartless as you get to know him, Gloria grows more lovable with time. Because Bear was affable and willing to listen to her at length on the telephone, he and Gloria got along well for nearly ten years, until he left Boston to become director of neuropsychiatry at the Vanderbilt University School of Medicine in Tennessee.

Even today, Gloria remains angry at Mark for the failed brain operation. "I shouldn't say it," she said, "but I'd like to operate on *his* brain! The thought that Dr. Mark couldn't destroy me makes me feel a little better." Many times she planned to sue him. "I don't know why I never made a lawsuit. I guess I decided that God will take care of that man."

Gloria is fortunate compared to the eight or more patients who underwent the procedure bilaterally, all of whom showed no long-term clinical improvement, and some of whom languish, unable to function normally, in psychiatric institutions. Initially, Mark and Ervin wrote, the operation reduced patients' anger and violence but not the frequency of their seizures. Of a typical patient who had the procedure bilaterally, the doctors wrote two years after surgery, "We did not achieve our goal of controlling her epileptic seizures; nonetheless, we did stop her rage attacks." The fact that the procedure often affected rage but not seizures suggested to Peter Rogert Breggin, a psychiatrist and opponent of psychosurgery, "a lack of association between the pacified aggression and the epileptic brain disease."

In the long run, Mark's psychosurgery, like the earlier frontal lobotomy, accomplished something quite different from what was intended: several patients suffered severe and incapacitating memory loss. "We didn't see successes," according to Kuehnle, who knew several of Mark's psychosurgery patients. Bear added that "the operation didn't work out. Mark *was* well intended: he had a sincere desire to help patients in distress; and he argued that the lesions he made were so small"—the size of a plum, as Mark put it—"that doing it bilaterally was okay. But in retrospect, the thinking was inadequate; the science wasn't profound. You can't take out the amygdala bilaterally without disastrous results," including serious difficulty in thinking, feeling, and remembering. "Destroying [the amygdala] to cure one 'symptom' such as violence," Breggin stated, "makes no more sense than bombing a railway center to stop one passenger on one train." Kaplan, who had done neuropsychological testing on some of Mark's patients, added, "That experiment with the amygdalotomies really went down the tubes. Mark and Ervin tried to make a case for the 'criminal brain,' and, boy, that went into disrepute fast. The surgery wasn't worth anything." Since the early 1970s, no bilateral amygdalotomies have been performed.

Several years after the bilateral amygdalotomies that Mark carried out, the families of several patients were unhappy with the procedure's long-term results. One family went so far as to sue Mark and Ervin, his collaborator in violence research, for malpractice. The patient, Leonard A. Kille, who prior to the operation was an engineer for Honeywell and Polaroid, had developed TLE seizures as a young adult after injuring his head. He gradually became paranoid and quick to anger. If a driver cut him off on the highway, he pursued the driver, forced him to the side of the road, and beat him up. If his wife seemed inattentive, he threw her and their children against a wall. After these attacks, which lasted only minutes, his behavior was reminiscent of Dostoevsky's after seizures: "He would be overcome with remorse and grief and sob as uncontrollably as he had raged," Mark and Ervin wrote. "He would then go to sleep for a half-hour or so and wake up feeling refreshed and eager to work."

To pinpoint the location of his brain discharge, Mark implanted electrodes in Kille's right and left amygdalas, where he had detected epileptic discharge on an EEG. For ten weeks Mark stimulated his brain, creating both seizures and feelings of relaxation that seemed to prevent the seizures from progressing. By regularly stimulating these relaxed feelings, Mark said, he kept the patient "rage free for nearly three months." Then, explaining that he couldn't stimulate Kille indefinitely, Mark suggested a bilateral amygdalotomy.

The patient initially consented, but then changed his mind. "He agreed to this suggestion while he was relaxed from . . . stimulation of the amygdala," Mark and Ervin wrote. "However, twelve hours later, when this effect had worn off," he "turned wild and unmanageable. The idea of anyone's making a destructive lesion in his brain enraged him." The doctors encouraged him for weeks, until he finally accepted the idea.

The bilateral procedure was performed at Massachusetts General Hospital during the winter of 1966–67, when Kille was in his thirties. Michael Crichton, a Harvard medical student who was present during portions of the lengthy procedure, was so affected by what he observed that he later wrote a novel based on it, *The Terminal Man*, which became a 1972 best-seller and a film. In Crichton's fictionalized account, Dr. John Ellis, a taut neurosurgeon with thick glasses and a limp, implants forty electrodes in the brain of a young engineer with TLE. Attached to the electrodes is a postage stamp-sized computer, embedded in the engineer's neck, through which Ellis can read electrical activity from and deliver electric shocks to the brain. Each time the brain gears up for a seizure, the computer sends an electric shock to the amygdala, aborting the seizure. The engineer's seizures consist of horrible smells, blackouts, nausea, and acts of directed aggression, such as assaulting a woman and beating up a much stronger man. This violent behavior, Ellis says in the novel, is "part of the disease" of TLE.

The real-life "terminal man," according to Mark and Ervin, had a typical reaction to the bilateral amygdalotomy: his rage seemed to have been reduced, but his seizures remained. In 1970 the doctors wrote that in the four years after the operation Kille "has not had a single episode of rage. He continues, however, to have an occasional epileptic seizure with periods of confusion and disordered thinking."

Confusion and disordered thinking were hardly the worst of Kille's problems following the operation, according to his mother, Helen Geis. Kille was partially paralyzed for months. He lost his short-term memory and was unable to work. He became delusional, believing that Mark and Ervin were "controlling his brain by electrodes placed in his head," a situation that during the operation had been the case. He became even more violent than before the surgery. In 1968, after fighting with police, he was admitted to a Veterans Administration hospital outside Boston, which declared him "totally disabled," and he became a permanent inpatient there. A year or two later, he attacked his father. "He was destroyed by that operation," his mother said. "He has been almost a vegetable since." His condition never improved. Twenty-five years after the operation, Helen Geis described the surgery and its aftermath as "a long, tragic affair. Doctors can destroy people and get away with it. At least that experiment has been stopped."

In 1973, alleging that the operation had "permanently incapacitated" her son, Geis sued Mark and Ervin for two million dollars. The suit stated that Kille, once described by doctors as a brilliant engineer, was now "of unsound and unbalanced mind and incompetent to handle his personal affairs," as well as "permanently deprived" of his ability to work. Because Kille's brain was being stimulated when his permission for the operation was sought, the doctors were charged with not having obtained his informed consent, by "failing to inform him fully and fairly as to the true nature of the procedures and all the risks involved and to provide an accurate statement of the probability that the procedures would cure or completely alleviate his diagnosed affliction." The suit also alleged that the doctors failed to protect Kille's privacy, because without his consent they had written about his life in *Violence and the Brain*.

The case received wide publicity and went to a jury trial in Boston in November 1978. During the trial, which lasted nearly three months, the doctors' Harvard colleagues, including Geschwind, testified on their behalf. Chorover, who as an expert witness for the plaintiff introduced the jury to the workings of the temporolimbic brain, said later that "no physicians from Boston would testify against Mark and Ervin because the medical community here is very tight." Because of the weight of expert testimony in their favor and the lack of explicit rules regarding patient consent for surgery in the 1960s, Mark and Ervin were in February 1979 cleared of charges of malpractice in their treatment of Kille.

This verdict, Chorover later observed, also rested on the true meaning of the term "malpractice." "To be found guilty of malpractice one must be found to have been doing something that people in your position would normally not do. Hard-working, ambitious young doctor-researchers like Mark and Ervin know they have to do research, so that was not evidence of malpractice, and the theory they advanced—that psychosurgery could alter behavior without ill effects—had been around for a long time. It may have been wrong and ill considered and without significant foundation, but it was not malpractice."

Despite the verdict, Mark and Ervin paid a price for their work in psychosurgery. Their colleagues rallied around them during the trial, but many are hesitant to be associated with them now. Mark and Ervin were "clobbered" by criticism, Bear explained. "They became lightning rods for anger about psychosurgery. The system clamped down on them. Ervin was told that his appointment at Harvard University and Massachusetts General Hospital would not be renewed, so he left," taking positions at UCLA and then McGill. Mark stayed in Boston, "but he lost his strong connection with Massachusetts General Hospital," and he was made chief of neurosurgery at Boston City Hospital just as Harvard disaffiliated itself with that hospital. During the 1970s, Boston hospitals disassociated themselves from bilateral amygdalotomies and from psychosurgery. By the late 1980s, the only psychosurgical procedure being performed in Boston, at Massachusetts General Hospital, was a cingulotomy, the unilateral removal of a part of the temporal lobe called the cingulate gyrus, a nerve bundle connecting the limbic system to the cortex. This operation occasionally reduces extreme aggression and has no apparent ill effects.

Today, most neurosurgeons agree that the physical underpinnings of personality are not sufficiently understood to justify psychosurgery. While few experts dispute that there are brain regions where a neurosurgeon with an electrode can provoke in anyone aggressive or sexual feelings, doctors doubt that surgically removing these places invariably removes or even alters the person's tendencies toward those traits. Lobotomy "is now considered an evolutionary throwback," Elliot Valenstein wrote in 1986, "akin more to the early practice of trepanning the skull to allow the demons to escape than to modern medicine." Like another treatment for TLE, the application of hot irons to the body, which was abandoned a century ago, the psychosurgical procedures that Mark used on Gloria and other TLE patients have fallen out of favor. In the 1980s, Paul MacLean, a physician who believed that doctors should not recommend elective procedures that they would not want done on themselves, asked surgeons meeting at the National Institutes of Health to raise their hands if they would be willing to have electrodes placed in their amygdalas. No one raised a hand.

Without the diagnosis of TLE, Mark would have had far more difficulty justifying psychosurgery on aggressive patients. "Epilepsy was sort of the excuse for using surgery to research Mark and Ervin's primary interest, which was personality," Chorover suggested. "At the trial, the doctors made a big thing about how they had operated for epilepsy, but in all their writings epilepsy is given fairly short shrift." TLE, with its fuzzy boundaries, its merging of body and mind, and its association with anger and personality change, lends itself to such questionable practices.

Although psychosurgery is no longer used for TLE, the standard unilateral temporal lobectomy continues to be offered to patients whose seizures do not respond well to other treatments. Gloria, with long-standing seizures and multiple epileptic focuses in both hemispheres, is not a candidate for this operation. Jill, however, is.

A young person with a recent diagnosis of seizures, Jill became a surgical candidate about two years after her diagnosis. Schomer raised the possibility of her having a temporal lobectomy during a meeting in his office, in 1983. He said that if her seizures continued to respond poorly to anticonvulsants and if her seizure focus could be found, surgery was "an option." Jill, who had never before heard of epilepsy surgery, was shocked. Her neurologist calmly explained that the operation has few ill effects, such as infection and bleeding; it is elective; and at least a year would pass before he would know if she was even a good candidate.

Jill's surgical workup began a year later, with her admission to Beth Israel Hospital for long-term EEG telemetry. "I'll be out awhile for a breast reduction and a fanny lift," she told colleagues before she departed her office for a six-week medical leave. She wanted no visitors, she affirmed. At the hospital for three weeks, she spent most of her time attached to an EEG and a video machine, which recorded both the underlying electrical activity and the clinical appearance of numerous seizures. Her head was wrapped in white bandages, which protected the electrodes glued to her scalp over her temporal lobes. To increase the frequency of her seizures, doctors ordered her to stay awake playing video games through the night. Their goal was to determine which hemisphere contained her seizure focus. In addition, they wondered if they might find EEG evidence of a slow-growing tumor, which is the worry of any neurologist whose patient develops epilepsy for unknown reasons as an adult. If present, a tumor would necessitate a different neurosurgical procedure: it would have to be removed.

Several weeks after Jill returned to work, Schomer called her at her office with the telemetry results. Her EEG reports were still ambiguous, he said. He had been unable to detect either a tumor or even the hemisphere in which her seizures started. Jill's reaction was dismay. She felt that the time in the hospital had been for naught. But when she told her colleague Ted, he cried, "Great news!"

"It isn't great news," she replied hotly. "I have the rest of my life taking drugs."

"You're lucky you don't have a golf ball growing in your head," he countered.

Jill might have preferred the golf ball. Her hospital roommate, another young woman with TLE, had been found to have a tumor, which had already been removed. Jill felt jealous. She was tired of drugs. "Sometimes," she said, "I wish my doctors would say something concrete like, 'We'll go in and take it out and you'll be all better.'" However awful, a tumor would at least reduce her options to one. There would be no more choices for her to make.

The next step in her surgical workup, Schomer explained, would be a more invasive diagnostic procedure, requiring a six-week hospital stay. A neurosurgeon would implant in both her temporal lobes depth electrodes, from which EEG readings could be taken from inside her brain over several weeks. Depth electrodes sometimes provide clearer readings of deep brain activity, so this procedure might answer Schomer's questions about the location of her seizure focus. On the other hand, it, too, might be inconclusive. Jill, who had had enough fiddling with her brain, decided to wait.

Like many people with chronic disorders, she denied the existence of her illness whenever she felt well. "TLE is always a nonissue when it isn't bothering me," she confessed. "Confronting it focuses too much on having seizures rather than on being healthy." As a result, her treatment advanced slowly. "If she feels well for three months," Spiers said, "she doesn't want to do anything about it. She gradually blossoms again, dating more and expanding her circle of friends. Then she feels bad for a couple of weeks, and she pulls back again."

In the meantime, her drug trials and occasional brain scans and EEGs continued, as her doctors monitored her changing condition. Because the brain scans were draining, time-consuming, and sometimes humiliating, Jill tended to avoid them as long as she could. The one she worked hardest to avoid was the magnetic resonance imaging scan, known as an MRI, which Schomer ordered once a year because it was designed to detect a slow-growing tumor that could press on her temporal lobes, causing TLE. Having an MRI involves lying completely still for an hour between two huge, parallel, doughnut-shaped magnets, each weighing twenty-two tons. The first time Jill went through it, she was fine. The next time, she left the medical center before the test was completed. Lying between the magnets, she had become claustrophobic, panicked, and screamed, "Pull me out!" until the technician halted the scanner and released her.

Ten months later, at Schomer's bidding, she finally returned to the MRI test center. To the cheerful technician who ushered her toward the test room she said playfully, "Taking bets on whether I'll make it this time?" She paused. "Just do the right part of my body so I don't have to come back!" Jill wore a loose sweatsuit and high-top sneakers. To help herself relax during the test, she had taken an extra dose of Xanax, an antianxiety medication that she frequently takes to help her face an impending seizure.

"You took *four* Xanax?" the technician, Donna, asked, aware that an ordinary dose is one pill. "How do you feel?"

"I feel mellow," Jill replied. Entering the test room, she passed a middle-aged man and his wife on their way out. "Even with two Valiums in me I still can't go through this test," he said, stricken. "I fought cancer for two years and I've had lots of CAT scans. But I can't do this."

Jill ignored him and entered the test room, its walls, floor, and ceiling a glossy white. Nearly filling it was a square, white machine with a fifteen-inch-high horizontal opening across its middle into which Jill would be slid. The manufacturer's name, "FONAR," was emblazoned in orange on the machine's plastic surface. Hidden inside the whiteness were the magnets, one above the slit and the other below. At waist level, a large metal prong supported a stretcher. Jill looked at the machine, took off her sweatshirt, and said, "I feel like I'm in Woody Allen's *Sleeper*."

The machine, a marvel of modern medical technology, had been called an NMR (for "nuclear magnetic resonance") when it became available about five years before. But the word *nuclear* had frightened patients, even though it referred not to power or bombs but to the nucleus, or center, of the atom; so the name had been changed. The MRI, which uses magnetism and radio waves to take pictures of human body parts, is similar to a CAT scan but safer, because it employs no radiation. It also provides clearer pictures of soft tissue, such as organs, than do CAT scans, which are preferred for producing images of bones. The machine's magnetic field is six thousand times stronger than the earth's gravitational pull, so that when a person lies inside it, the hydrogen protons in her body stand on end. Then the machine emits a sudden pulse of radio frequency matching the frequency of the protons' spin, which knocks them flat. Once the pulse is over, the protons, like soldiers that have been shot, stand back up, each at a rate dependent on their tissue's structure and density. Protons in bone rise more quickly than protons in soft tissue, and those in cancer rise more slowly. As the protons rise, they resonate, emitting echoes. The machine measures the radio frequency of the echo, transforms it into a digital signal, and sends it into the adjoining control room, where it appears as a photographic image on a computer screen.

Jill sat on the edge of the stretcher. "Take off that hair clip," Donna ordered.

"It's plastic," Jill said. From her last visit she knew to leave her watch and earrings at home, away from the machine's pull. A small coin or implanted metal screw would probably cause no harm, but Donna reminds people to remove all metal. One man had a pen she didn't know about. When the machine was turned on, the pen emerged from his pocket and floated, in alignment with the magnetic field, between the magnet and his face.

Jill lay back on the stretcher. Donna arranged strips of foam around her head and covered it with a fiberglass arc, like a blindfold, that contained copper coils through which the radio pulse would come. She pressed a button marked PRESET SCAN CENTER to take the machine's aim at the center of Jill's brain. A red light shone on Jill's face. "Close your eyes," Donna said, "because I've got the laser on you." She reminded Jill of the necessity of staying still throughout the test. "It's going to be real loud in there," she warned, tapping the machine with her fingernails to imitate the sound of the radio pulse. Jill took another half of a Xanax from a pillbox in her pocket and vowed, "I'm *not* going to have to come back this year and do this again."

Donna pressed the bed-control button. The stretcher and Jill rose to the level of the space between the magnets. By hand, Donna slid the stretcher back into the machine. Jill's head was at the center of the machine, her body hardly visible. Only her pink socks could be seen.

The Xanax had worked. She felt strange and silly, but calm. Keeping her eyes shut helped: it enabled her to pretend she was somewhere else. If she was lucky, she thought, she would fall asleep.

"Bend your knees. Get more comfortable," Donna told her. "What kind of music do you like?"

"What have you got?" Jill asked, pleased to have a choice in this controlled environment.

"Classical, pop, jazz . . . " Jill chose classical, and Donna moved toward the control room. At the door she stopped to look back. "Put your arms out," she said. Jill rustled her arms listlessly. Donna shouted, "Out!" Finally she cried, "Like a crucifix!" and left the room.

"This is really bizarre," Jill muttered to herself. "Here I am like Jesus Christ in this two-million-dollar machine."

In the control room, Donna pressed a button that summoned a muffled recording of Handel's *Water Music*. Into her keyboard she punched instructions for the first series of photographic slices of Jill's brain. Computerized parameters appeared on the screen: "Number of slices," "Number of images per slice." Donna watched Jill through a window cut into the wall. Through an intercom, she asked, "You hear rumbling?"

"Yes," came the faint reply, carried by a microphone near Jill's head.

"This next set's going to be a little louder," Donna said.

In the test room, Jill barely heard her. The machine produced a sound like the deep static thunder of broken stereo speakers, punctuated by loud, rapid-fire clicks. Jill breathed deeply and tuned the noises out. She meditated. Eventually she slept, her hands folded, as the machine hummed.

In the control room, away from the noise, Donna watched a pair of images of Jill's brain slide across a computer screen every few seconds. Some sections pictured slices of her brain as viewed from the side, and others pictured slices as viewed from the front. In all of them, a ribbon of gray matter surrounded the rounded mass of white matter; nerve cell bodies, which lie at the surface of the human brain, look gray, while their dendrites, the stringy appendages connecting them to other neurons, look white. At the end of the session, Donna punched buttons to summon a picture of Jill's temporal lobes.

"All done!" she shouted, rushing into the test room to pull the stretcher out.

Jill rubbed the sleep from her eyes as she emerged from between the magnets. "I was in there an hour?" she asked.

"Yup. Did you hear the clicking?"

"I only heard the music. Now I know the trick to having this test: take drugs and listen to music!" Before leaving the room, she asked Donna, "Did you find anything weird in there?" She pointed at her head. "Anything growing?"

"You know I can't tell you what I see," Donna said.

Jill sighed and headed for the waiting area where she had arrived three hours earlier. Soon a receptionist handed her a huge brown envelope. Jill opened it and gazed at the black-and-white prints of her eyeballs, her internal auditory canals, and her brain, which looked to her like images of crabs. Another set would be sent to Schomer.

On the street outside the test center, she breathed in the muddy smell of spring. She clutched her packet of MRI photos and thought, absurdly, of hanging them on her office wall. Giddy and exhausted, she shouted, "I did it! I won't be afraid of it again!" She recalled Schomer's eagerness for her to have this test, and anticipated his pleasure once he knew about it. He would soon tell her that the MRI results indicated nothing out of the ordinary growing in her head. A smudge on an artery that might have been an aneurism would turn out to be of no concern.

This negative bad news is a kind of good news, the kind that Jill generally gets. In the early years after her diagnosis, her weeks and hours were devoted to learning negative facts, ruling awful things out of her life, which left little time to rule positive things in. After the MRI she was back where she had started. Since the chance remained that a yet-undetected tumor caused her seizures, in a year she would have to return for another MRI, and yet another every year after that. At times, Jill thought, TLE had turned her life into a treadmill and forced her to put many choices aside, foremost among them committing herself to a life partner and possibly having a child. "Some days, all I can do when I get home from work is crawl into bed," she said. "When I'm feeling sick, I can't think about anyone but myself, so how could I have a committed relationship or care for a baby?" Ever-present was the unpleasant question of surgery, which, if she decided to pursue it, would mean putting everything else on hold for two more years. Life with TLE was rather like Wonderland, in Lewis Carroll's *Through the Looking-Glass*, in which effects are altered and decisions are infinitely delayed. As the Queen tells Alice, who has asked why she doesn't move even though she is running as fast as she can, "Here, you see, it takes all the running you can do, to stay in the same place."

About five years after her diagnosis, when she was thirty-six, Jill debarked from the treadmill of TLE. Like Flaubert, who had abandoned the treatments proposed by his father and turned to the task of becoming a writer, Jill decided to take charge of her own care. She resolved "to stop obsessing about TLE and try to get control of my life." She determined, first, to improve her overall health. Once a chain smoker, she gave up cigarettes. She stopped taking cocaine, which she had used since a friend offered it to her a year or so after her diagnosis. Finding that the drug elevated her mood, cleared her head, and relieved her headaches, Jill had developed a habit, sometimes taking as much as a gram of cocaine in an evening, to the dismay of Spiers, who warned her that despite its apparent palliative effects, cocaine is addictive and causes numerous health problems, including seizures. In another change, Jill cut most fat and sugar from her diet. She made sure to get enough sleep and began rising at six every morning in order to jog two miles. For the first time in her life, she exercised regularly. To unwind and relax at the end of the workday, she signed up for a sculpture course at an art school.

Besides these life-style changes, Jill made a decision regarding the surgery for TLE. After months of tossing around the idea of returning to the hospital for EEG monitoring with implanted electrodes, she determined that unless her condition worsened, she would not pursue the surgical workup. "In my heart of hearts," she said, the words spilling out, "I don't want to have the surgery, because I'm going to lose. It would take two or three years of my life and I honestly believe I would never be the same. I wouldn't be *me*. I mean, you can't have your matter just scraped out of your head and be the same person. The doctors don't even know what's in the part of your brain that they remove. There's a chance I could be better, but that chance is only one in three." The postsurgical patients that Jill had seen in Schomer's waiting area, with their shaven, gauze-covered heads, all seemed far sicker than she. She had actually met only one of these patients, a younger woman who had had a temporal lobectomy at eighteen. Spiers had asked Jill to help this woman find a job. "Now, she's *fine*, Jill," Spiers had said, knowing that Jill would expect the woman to be odd. But the woman had confirmed Jill's expectation by being sticky. "She called me three times in two hours," Jill said, "and that's just not normal!"

Spiers, who predicted that because of Jill's inconsistent response to drugs "she is headed for surgery eventually," agreed with her assessment that she had a choice. "Either she can focus on living, or she can focus on being sick," he said. "She's got to go ahead and live her life, or she's got to put her life on hold and proceed with the surgical workup. That second option is not a great treat for anybody, certainly not one who, as Jill would perceive herself, has a lot to lose. She lives in an apartment on Beacon Hill, she has friends, she has a responsible job with power and prestige, and she gets paid to make decisions about other people's lives."

Around the time that Jill decided against pursuing the surgical option, her condition began to improve for reasons her doctors could not fully explain. Mysteriously, five hundred milligrams of Tegretol, an anticonvulsant that her doctors had already tried in various doses by itself and with other drugs, seemed to do what no other anticonvulsant had done before: consistently reduce the number of her seizures. Her seizures did not stop altogether, but the flashes of colors, the periodic dizziness, and the occasional feeling of being lost in a familiar place all occurred far less often than before. Most important, the panic attacks now came only once every six to twelve months, usually just before she menstruated. At this frequency, seizures were no longer a major worry for Jill.

Her life was far from perfect—she still had to take Tegretol daily and have occasional EEGs and annual MRIs—but she had found a new stability. Once frustrated that the disorder controlled her, she had now found ways of incorporating TLE and its treatment into her life, taking control where she could, and accepting those realms in which she could not. "I've managed a way to function with TLE," she said with quiet pride, "so it's no longer a big part of my life. I can tell people about my TLE now. I'm not embarrassed by it anymore. I feel so far away from where I was a few years ago." Although her TLE had not gone away, its worst effects seemed to have passed.

The reasons for Jill's improvement are not clear. The life-style changes she made, her decision to discontinue the surgical workup, and possible changes in hormonal, chemical, or electrical activity in her brain may all be factors in her new state. Jill's situation is not unusual among people with TLE. No treatment method has been found to work consistently, and doctors are often unable to explain why a patient suddenly feels better or worse. Today, as in the past, the route to successful treatment of TLE remains a mystery.

CHAPTER SEVEN

Body and Mind

On the sunroof of her apartment on Beacon Hill, Jill sits on a wooden stool, her face fixed in concentration. This sunny Tuesday afternoon, she is at home, having resigned from her job. No longer captive to silk and pearls, she wears old sneakers and jeans, a paisley bandana around her head, and thick suede gloves without fingertips. She wields a power chisel; its black cord snakes across the gravel roof, amid potted herbs, into a window of her apartment. Before her, on a square stand, is the object of her concentration, a block of white Carrara marble.

After nearly twenty years as a personnel director, Jill is now a sculptor. Like van Gogh, who abruptly in his late twenties developed an "excessive sensitivity" to the visual world, Jill in her mid–thirties felt a powerful urge to become an artist. Other than the obligatory ceramics course at childhood summer camp, she had never before participated in the arts. To satisfy her new desire, she called local art schools and signed up for a beginning course in clay sculpture. The next semester, she took an intermediate course and quickly moved to her chosen medium, stone. Before long, she was devoting every free hour to her art. Each evening after work, she changed her clothes and walked to an open studio at the art school, where she worked simultaneously on several abstract marble sculptures. "I have the same passion about sculpture that I once had about directing personnel," she said, amazed. "I never thought about sculpture before, but now I think about it all the time. I get really excited when I see a piece of stone: I want to feel it, look at it, make something beautiful from it. I have so many ideas."

Now, two years after beginning art classes and eight years after her seizures started, Jill is "the happiest I've ever been," she says as she wipes a streak of white marble dust from her brow. To support her new life-style, she occasionally takes part-time consulting jobs in personnel. Not long ago, dipping into the savings account that Spiers had encouraged her to start, she traveled to Carrara, Italy, to study with a master artisan. In an outdoor studio with views of the Alps and the Adriatic Sea, Jill sculpted eleven hours a day for three months. Toward the end of her stay in Italy, she purchased sculpting equipment and nine hundred kilos of white and pink Italian marble, which she had shipped to her apartment in Boston. There she continues the daily regimen she began in Italy. She works on her sunroof in the warm months and in a rented studio during the winter. While she intends to submit her work to galleries, she has no illusions about the likelihood of supporting herself with her art.

Although Jill hates to think that her disorder abrogates her personal will, she believes that her sudden change of career is related to her TLE. "With TLE, I see things slightly differently than before," she explains. "I have visions and images that normal people don't have. Some of my seizures"—the out-of-body experiences, intensified colors, and floating sensations—"are like entering another dimension, the closest to religion or spiritual feelings that I've ever had. Epilepsy has given me a rare vision and insight into myself, and sometimes beyond myself, and it has played to my creative side. Without TLE, I would not have begun to sculpt."

Experts agree that her new vocation most likely has a neuropsychological cause. "Jill's abrupt switch to sculpture may well be a form of hypergraphia, the right-hemisphere corollary of the left-temporal-lobe epileptics who write a lot," Kaplan says. The neuropsychologist speculates that changes in seizure activity caused Jill to move from the personnel field to sculpture. The aptitude for both types of work is mediated by the brain's right hemisphere—personnel management by frontotemporal structures, and sculpture by occipitotemporoparietal regions controlling visual-spatial skills. According to Kaplan, if Jill's seizures started in her left hemisphere, as her doctors suspect, epileptic activity may have switched hemispheres over the years, spawning a "mirror focus" in the rear of the right hemisphere and over-stimulating visual-spatial areas there. Or if her suspected prenatal brain damage was bilateral, abnormal activity in the right hemisphere may have developed only recently into seizures, causing her at the same time to pursue the highly spatial activity of sculpture. In another possible scenario, preexisting right-sided seizure activity may have moved from the front to the back of the hemisphere, altering her right-hemisphere skills. Alternatively, Tegretol may have reduced right-hemisphere seizure activity, enabling the ordinary activity of regions controlling visual-spatial skills to emerge. Bear agrees with Kaplan that Jill's sculpting is consistent with Geschwind's syndrome. While her suspected left-hemisphere seizure focus differentiates her from the four TLE patients with visual-spatial hypergraphia whom the psychiatrist studied, it does not preclude her from manifesting "noteworthy artistic creativity." In fact, Bear notes, her "structural superiority of the right temporoparietal area" is likely to enhance her visual-spatial skills.

Without solving the puzzle of human creativity, the study of TLE indicates that abnormal brain activity plays a role in the making of art. Epilepsy, sometimes called "the poet's affliction," has affected not only ordinary artists like Jill and the celebrated authors and mystics cited by Bear but also numerous other famous people. The neurologist William Gordon Lennox viewed as epileptic the writers Petrarch, Tasso, and Dickens, the musicians Handel and Paganini, the religious figures Saint Cecilia and the Buddha, the philosophers Socrates, Pascal, and Swedenborg, the political leaders Julius Caesar, Richelieu, and Napoleon, the mathematician Pythagoras, and the scientist Isaac Newton. Other commentators have found evidence of epilepsy in Alexander the Great, Molière, Peter the Great, Eugène Delacroix, Rasputin, August Strindberg, and the actor Richard Burton.

While organic mental disorders like TLE are often assumed to produce "failures in intellectual function," according to Geschwind, "TLE with behavioral change is compatible with a distinctly superior level of intellectual performance." Bear adds that other disorders, such as schizophrenia, manic-depressive illness, and confusional states—which cause people to see the world in new and often bizarre ways, sometimes leading to artistic flights—can result in behavior that "might, in the broadest sense, be called creative." But these disorders impair other crucial functions. "While disruptions of the normal stream of thought result in improbable associations," Bear explains, "patients suffering from them typically lack the critical scrutiny or persistence of attention necessary to produce significant creative products." TLE is different from these disorders, because it spares essential functions like attention, concentration, and critical judgment, all of which are necessary to sustain artistry. At the same time, TLE predisposes people to such aspects of creative thinking as sensitivity, the ability to detect connections, and flexibility. The combination of these two factors, unique to this form of epilepsy, may even intensify the ability to see artistically and to transform that vision into art, Bear adds, because the disorder generates "intense motivation leading to sustained rather than fragmentary attention while preserving the essential faculty of critical judgment."

The brain mechanism underlying this remarkable effect remains unknown. Since the syndrome occurs independently from seizures, it is thought that the personality changes and the electrical storms share a cause, perhaps a physical or chemical abnormality that produces excess electrical activity in the emotional brain. Even more mysterious is the cause of hypergraphia in people who do not have TLE. No one has yet attempted to pinpoint the differences between the brain activity of a nonepileptic artist and the brain activity of an artist with TLE. Lacking data on the electrical activity of artists as they work, researchers can only speculate as to the relationship between artistic imagination and the disordered brain.

The relationship between other traits of Geschwind's syndrome and the same traits in nonepileptics is equally unclear. In time, however, because of the association between TLE and hyperreligiosity, this disorder may open the door to a scientific understanding of morality and religion. In the view of Leonard Katz, a professor of philosophy, the notion that TLE underlies the moral fervor of Charlie, Gloria, Dostoevsky, and van Gogh suggests that morality has an organic basis. "The fact that TLE patients are filled with intense gratitude and hypermoralism, characteristics considered a basis of morality," Katz notes, "confirms the suspicion that morality has a physiological substrate, which is probably dispersed throughout the limbic system of social animals like ourselves." Similarly, as the physician Macdonald Critchley pointed out, it is difficult to distinguish between TLE seizures and common mystical and religious states, all of which include flashes of light, incorporeal voices, and visions. Spiers surmises that everyone infrequently experiences seizure states like *déjà vu*, the feeling of a presence, or hallucinatory voices or visions, and that this mild, undiagnosed TLE in the general population may account for the widespread interest in mysticism, reincarnation, out-of-body experiences, UFOs, and aliens. The Canadian neurologist Persinger goes even further in associating TLE and religious states, saying that all spiritual experience derives from altered temporolimbic electrical activity. In Persinger's view, religion is our explanation for the feelings produced by this abnormal electrical activity. Most commentators agree that if TLE is at the root of moral fervor or religious states, its presence does not detract from their reality. As William James stated, it is "quite illogical . . . to plead the organic causation of a religious state of mind . . . in refutation of its claim to possess superior spiritual value." No medical condition can diminish the achievements of Flaubert, Tennyson, Maupassant, Muhammad, Moses, or Saint Paul.

Not all effects of TLE on personality and emotion are potentially as beneficial to society as the intensification of the drive to behave morally or spiritually or to create art. The incidence of TLE in violent criminals is also suprisingly high. While doctors have traditionally implicated psychosocial, genetic, and hormonal factors in violent behavior, they now also consider neurophysiological factors such as brain injury and neurological disease, which are currently believed to be the most common causes of explosive rage. In a study of violent psychiatric patients, as many as 94 percent showed evidence of brain damage. In another study, every one of twenty-nine death-row inmates had suffered head trauma, a common cause of seizure disorders. A different study of fourteen juvenile males on death row found that all had suffered serious head injuries as children, most had abnormal electrical activity in the brain, and several had seizures involving dizziness, *déjà vu*, and hallucinatory tastes and smells. The psychiatrist Dorothy Otnow Lewis, who carried out some of these studies, says that many violent people have a "limbic-psychotic-aggressive syndrome," a frequently unrecognized condition "on the border of psychiatry and neurology" consisting of temporolimbic seizures without an abnormal EEG. According to doctors, the EEGs of these patients may be negative because the technique is not sensitive to deep temporolimbic activity or because their seizures are not sufficiently intense to be measured. While the incidence of EEG abnormalities in the general population is estimated at only 15 percent, "between 50 and 75 percent of violent individuals have EEG abnormalities, often in the temporal lobes," according to Khoshbin. In fact, many doctors now believe that when a person suddenly and uncharacteristically commits a violent act, TLE should be considered as a possible cause.

These connections between violence and epilepsy have ramifications for both medicine and the law. On occasion, lawyers win verdicts of not guilty by reason of insanity on behalf of people with TLE accused of crimes, based on the assumption that a person is not responsible for acts committed during seizures. Doctors infrequently attempt to "treat" violence with anticonvulsant drugs. Khoshbin, for instance, has used Tegretol "with very good results" in nonepileptic patients with histories of violence and brain-scan evidence of abnormal temporal-lobe activity. Some researchers believe that further study of the links between epilepsy and violence may reopen the psychosurgery debate. Vernon Mark's position that violence can be reduced by changing certain regions of the brain "may turn out to be right," according to Spiers, who believes that surgeons may someday have the capacity, if not the discretion, to alter specific emotions and traits—rage, dread, sexual desire, religious feeling, even affability—by removing parts of the brain.

Unlike most diseases, TLE is associated with positive as well as negative experiences. But it is unknown why Geschwind's syndrome sometimes appears to advantage, as in Charlie, who is distinguished by his intellectual focus and pervasive, purposeful calm. The effects of the syndrome may reflect the preexisting personality, the location or extent of seizure activity, or the nature of the brain damage underlying the seizures. As Bear and others note, patients with epileptic scars in the right hemisphere of the brain display intense emotions, while patients with left-hemisphere scars are often sober, moral intellectuals.

The range of personality seen with TLE suggests a continuum between the abnormal and the normal. In all of us, passions, interest in religion and philosophy, and the drive to create may be anatomically based. After studying shyness and gregariousness in infants, the psychologist Jerome Kagan concluded that such personality traits are inborn, rather than acquired. In his research he found that each personality type was associated with physical characteristics: shy infants tended to be tall, thin, and blue-eyed, while gregarious babies were generally brown-eyed mesomorphs. In response to the stress of an unfamiliar situation, shy infants had hearts that beat faster than those of gregarious infants, a difference that Kagan attributed to slight differences in the amygdala and hippocampus, limbic structures that control heart rate, muscle tension, and release of stress hormones. Similarly, Minnesota psychologists found that identical twins reared apart were on average as similar in personality as identical twins who were raised together, suggesting a genetic or structural basis for personality. According to Spiers, every individual has some brain damage, usually too subtle to appear on an ordinary EEG, and the location and extent of this damage is frequently linked to her proclivities. The stereotypical absentminded professor, for instance, who recalls details of her discipline but cannot locate her glasses, may have slight damage in her right hemisphere that caused her other hemisphere to overcompensate, enhancing her verbal and analytical skills. "People may not like to hear it, because it seems predetermined," Spiers says, "but the reason I'm analytical, I write a lot, I'm very right-handed, and I'm not particularly athletic is probably that I'm strongly left-hemisphere-dominant. And I'm probably left-hemisphere-dominant because my right hemisphere is a little damaged. Clearly, parts of my brain didn't develop as well as others. Now it doesn't represent a dysfunction in my case, but it's there. The fact is, all human behaviors are controlled by the brain."

TLE provides a key to the association between brain and behavior because of "the number of other strangenesses—left-

handedness, autoimmune disorders, and hormonal alterations—that run along with it," Spiers adds. "Sometimes the
same things that cause epilepsy result in giftedness. If you damage an area early enough in life, the corresponding area on the
other side has a chance to overdevelop." At the time of his
death, Geschwind was engaged in research on the confluence of
unusual skills and brain abnormalities. Working with the pro-
prietor of a shop in London that specializes in objects for left-
handers, Geschwind and a colleague found that left-handed
people, who constitute about 15 percent of the population, tend
to excel in right-hemisphere-led fields such as architecture, theoretical mathematics, and physics, and that they have a high
incidence of stuttering, prematurely gray hair, hormonal irregularities, and such disorders as dyslexia, autoimmune diseases,
and migraine headaches—all disorders that occur with increased frequency in people with TLE. Geschwind theorized
that these clustered tendencies stem from brain changes caused
by the prenatal influence of the hormone testosterone, which
affects the growth of the brain and the immune system. The
same testosterone-induced brain changes may also underlie
some cases of TLE. Another possibility is that certain families
carry a gene for epilepsy, such as the gene molecular biologists
have already found in mice. While no clear Mendelian pattern
of inheritance has been demonstrated in human epilepsy, studies show an unusually high incidence of seizures or EEG abnormalities in close relatives of people with TLE.

Because TLE shows that specific changes in behavior result
from corresponding physical changes in the brain, this disorder
has become an important avenue for research into the organic
basis of personality. In recent years, as doctors realized the ramifications of Geschwind's syndrome even for people who do not
have TLE, their reluctance to discuss it has begun to fall away.
Defining hypergraphia, hyperreligiosity, rage, and altered sexuality as features of a disorder with an organic basis, rather than as
results of a flawed will, has changed how doctors respond to the
traits. Geschwind wrote not long before his death, "Behavioral
change in TLE deserves very special consideration, since it is
probably the only cause of major change in behavior for which
we have a plausible mechanism of pathogenesis. . . . The importance of this syndrome results from its clinical fascination, its

frequency, and . . . its unique capacity to present to us a clear-cut physiological paradigm for the occurrence of behavioral change after alterations in the brain."

This is what intrigues contemporary brain researchers the most about TLE—the fact that it demonstrates the interconnectedness of physiology and personality. In this respect, the disorder contributes to the growing rapprochement between neurology and psychiatry, the two medical specialties dealing with human behavior, which until recently functioned largely independently. Neurology and psychiatry seemed practically indistinguishable at their beginning in the nineteenth century. Sigmund Freud, the founder of psychiatry and himself a neurologist, said in 1891, "We must recollect that all our provisional ideas in psychology will presumably one day be based on an organic substructure." Yet the disciplines rapidly grew apart, dividing up their common turf: brain and mind. By the early twentieth century, most neurologists explored the brain's structure, noting patients' paralysis, gait disturbances, strokes, spinal-cord damage, and other physical signs, while psychiatrists explored the mind, noting patients' recollections and feelings. As the psychiatrist D. W. Winnicott described this forced separation of brain and mind in 1919, "The brain is the mass of gray and white matter which lies hidden in the skull, whereas the mind is that part of a person which stores memories, thinks and wills (if it does will at all). The brain is unlike the mind as a nerve is unlike the impulse that travels down it."

In dividing brain and mind, the medical specialties solidified a distinction reflected in etymology and in post-Renaissance philosophy. In Greek, *neuron* means "nerve" or "sinew," while *psyche* means "soul" or "mind," so that *neurology* is literally "talking about nerves," whereas *psychiatry* means "talking about the mind." In addition, modern science proceeded from the belief in a dichotomy of body and mind described in 1637 by the French mathematician and philosopher René Descartes. "The intelligent nature is distinct from the corporeal," Descartes wrote in *Discourse on Method*, "so that 'I,' that is to say, the mind by which I am what I am, is wholly distinct from the body." For Descartes, mind was not a function of the brain, but a separate "nonphysical" substance. Descartes's theory, which was called "dualism" because it assumed the dual natures of body and mind, established the modern chasm between mental and physical states, and it opened the way for rational, scientific thought by conceiving of a separation between the physical and spiritual worlds. It also established the "mind-body problem"—how mind and body relate to each other—"the ultimate of ultimate problems," according to William James. Descartes's solution was to say that the mind guides the body as a pilot steers a ship.

In medicine, for the most part, dualism became the rule. Most doctors were taught to conceive of physical disorders and personality as separate categories, which accounts for Stephen Waxman's initial amazement at Geschwind's suggestion that specific behavioral changes might have a distinct anatomical base. As a result of the institutional division between brain and mind, the neurologist Michael Gazzaniga notes, many twentieth-century "brain scientists and mind scientists could not talk to each other. Each . . . laid undue claim to understanding the mind-brain function from his own perspective alone. Let's say you have a delusional friend who thinks he is the King of Siam. The conventional brain scientist says the problem with your friend is biochemical, and the conventional mind scientist notes something about a traumatic childhood. Both ideas . . . miss the mark . . . by a mile." Similarly, according to Kaplan, if a patient who was shown a standard line drawing of an ice tong said he saw "a coffin," a psychiatrist might interpret this error as a sign that the patient was depressed, while a neurologist might view it as a sign of a right-hemisphere lesion causing the patient to neglect the entire left side of space; "the right half of the drawing of the ice tong *does* look like a coffin," Kaplan explains.

The demise of composer and pianist George Gershwin is another example of doctors' difficulties in distinguishing between the neurological and the psychiatric. Edwards recalls that when Gershwin was in his thirties his performances began to be punctuated with fifteen-second pauses. Doctors simply recommended that he reduce his stress. Soon afterward, Gershwin fell into a coma and died. At his autopsy a large tumor was discovered in his right temporal lobe. The tumor had hemorrhaged, causing his death, and it had also caused his pauses, which, according to Edwards, were seizures. The psychological misdiagnosis of "stress" prevented the neurological diagnosis.

In the 1960s, with the rise of behaviorism, the waning of

strict Freudianism in psychiatry, and the success of new drugs in treating the symptoms of psychiatric diseases such as schizophrenia, depression, and manic-depressive illness, the division between neurology and psychiatry began to break down. Experts suspected that many conditions once thought to be either neurological or psychiatric are in fact both. Geschwind, who was convinced that brain cannot be separated from behavior, or body from mind, attempted to further their merger by founding a neurological subspecialty uniting psychology and physiology; in 1978, at Beth Israel Hospital in Boston, he opened the first behavioral neurology unit in the country.

By the late 1980s, according to Gazzaniga, scientists were "beginning to understand how the brain and mind interact." Coming from a variety of disciplines called "neurosciences," researchers increasingly saw mind and body as not separate but interdependent, each having some control. "A rigid, narrowly physical or psychologic approach always proves to be inadequate and must be supplanted by a broader psychobiologic one," asserts the most recent edition of the standard neurology textbook. The challenge now, Gazzaniga adds, is "to come up with a conceptual framework that can tie together abnormalities of brain tissue, or, more commonly, normal variations in brain chemistry, with the personal, psychological reality of our individual minds." Gradually, as Geschwind predicted, the "no-man's-land" between neurology and psychiatry has become a "common ground."

TLE, a "neuropsychiatric" disorder with physiological causes and psychological effects, has become the preeminent disorder of this borderland. Geschwind considered TLE "a useful model for the major psychoses, because of its association with dysfunction at specific loci in the central nervous system." Psychosis and major depression occur about fifteen times as often in people with TLE as in the general population. For unknown reasons, schizophrenia tends to appear with left-hemisphere epileptic lesions, while manic-depressive illness and depression are more common in patients with right-hemisphere lesions. TLE and psychiatric disorders share symptoms, such as disembodied voices, visions, exaggerated emotions, and bizarre and inexplicable behavior. Many schizophrenics have abnormalities in their temporal lobes. It is not clear how many other psychiatric conditions, from obsessive-compulsive behavior to panic disorder, may be biologically based.

Increasingly, doctors suspect that neurological disease underlies psychiatric disorders. "Disease of the brain is an important and often treatable cause of behavior disorders ... in psychiatry," Geschwind said, noting that 30 percent of patients first admitted to mental hospitals turned out to be suffering from neurological disorders. Because of the potential for misdiagnosis of TLE and other neurological disorders, contemporary psychiatric evaluations include an initial neurological examination, often including sophisticated brain scans, to rule out neurological causes for apparently psychiatric conditions. According to Nancy Andreasen, a psychiatrist, mental illness is caused by biochemical, neuroendocrine, structural, and genetic abnormalities. Major "psychiatric" disorders like schizophrenia and manic-depressive illness probably belong within the realm of neurology, adds the psychiatrist E. Fuller Torrey. Stephen Signer, a neuropsychiatrist, writes, "The current approach of neuropsychiatrists, neuropsychologists, and behavioral neurologists regards behavioral disorders (mood disorders, psychosis, certain types of personality change, etc.) as a product of change in, by, and of the brain. This redefinition should lead not to a denial of the reality or burden of these illnesses, but to remove their stigma." Going even further than these physicians, Spiers contends that every condition described in the diagnostic manual of psychiatry "can be due to either epilepsy or some other neurological illness. Even if only half of all psychiatric patients" are being misdiagnosed and mistreated, he adds, this poses "a big problem" for doctors in the assessment of psychiatric disease.

Because TLE crosses the traditional boundary between psychiatry and neurology, improved methods of recognizing and treating it may lead to a revolution in the diagnosis and treatment of psychiatric disorders. According to Geschwind's colleague M-Marsel Mesulam, TLE is "the royal road to understanding the organic basis" of psychiatric disease. The disorder holds forth hope of advancing knowledge in both neurology and psychiatry and leading to a better understanding of the physiological causes of mental illness and mental health.

Much of the current research into TLE is devoted to diagnosis, with the greatest emphasis on improving the methods of detecting seizure activity or underlying brain damage. Recent decades have brought new diagnostic tools such as PET (positron emission tomography) scans, which display the relative activity of various brain regions, CAT scans, and MRIs. These techniques, however, are expensive and still not widely used, and for diagnosing TLE no machine has replaced the EEG. Yet the traditional EEG has significant drawbacks. Large and cumbersome, it is available only within major medical centers. It produces a vast amount of data—in twenty-four hours, several miles of paper that, when stacked, stands nearly four feet high—most containing no seizure activity both because seizure focuses are often inaccessible to electrodes and because patients typically seize only about once a week. Since EEG abnormalities usually occur without the patient's conscious awareness and apart from any apparent clinical change, patients are unable to alert doctors in advance. Extraneous electrical activity caused by bodily movements, called artifact, often makes the EEG difficult to read.

John Ives, a soft-spoken biomedical engineer from Toronto who has held academic appointments at both the Montreal Neurological Institute and a Harvard-affiliated hospital in Boston, spends his days trying to solve such problems. In 1972, using off-the-shelf computer components, he developed a long-term EEG monitoring system that could monitor a hospitalized patient for weeks. By 1980 Ives had developed an ambulatory outpatient monitoring system. A portable, battery-pack EEG machine with a forty-megabyte hard disk that holds four hours of EEG recordings, it can be worn over the patient's shoulder like a purse. The machine's recorder can be turned on either by the patient, who, if she feels a seizure coming, can push the Record button, or by the machine itself, which, if it detects abnormal EEG activity, automatically stores the ongoing activity as well as the previous two minutes. To deal with the massive amount of data produced by the ordinary EEG, Ives programmed a DEC VAX computer to scan the pages, pinpointing abnormalities. To reduce the amount of artifact in EEG recordings, he attached a miniature amplifier to a large noncomputerized inpatient EEG. The amplifier can be worn on the patient's head.

Research into the diagnosis of TLE has the additional benefit of raising new possibilities for treatment. For instance, as doc-

tors' ability to detect the exact location of the brain lesions leading to EEG abnormalities improves, the success rate of the
surgery also improves. "To take out epileptic brain tissue," Ives
says, "you need accuracy" in localizing seizure activity, "and that
requires high-powered technology." Since Ives became a mem-
ber of the epilepsy surgery team at Beth Israel Hospital in 1983,
the hospital has been able to work up more patients for the operation. "Now we work up one to two a week, about fifty percent of
whom go to surgery," Ives says. "We look for patients with clear
focal abnormal activity. A few years ago, before we had [this]
long-term EEG monitoring that can catch actual seizures, all
surgical decisions were based on interictal activity," which is far
less precise.

Ives's inventions may have applications to forms of treatment
other than surgery. For instance, he envisions programming a
computerized EEG to detect the early signs of a patient's
"seizure signature," a unique EEG pattern that occurs only during seizures. The machine could then warn the patient of the
incipient seizure. "Presently, there's nothing in the EEG that tells
us that the patient is going to seize in twenty minutes. Sometimes we detect the onset of a seizure in the focus a few seconds
in advance, and if we tell the patient that he's about to have a
seizure, he is sometimes able to stop it consciously by, say, grab-
bing his arm, which may be some kind of negative feedback."

The engineer also anticipates further miniaturization of the
computerized EEG so that it can be mounted on, or even inside,
a patient. "If electrodes could be placed in an area of the brain
where seizure onset can be detected," he says, "a suggestion"—
an electric current—"could be fed back to the patient internally,"
in the hope of preventing the seizure. "It could all be purely
automatic, like a cardiac pacemaker, which detects a low heart
rate and gives the heart an extra pulse. In such a feedback system, the patient might not even be aware of the suggestion." This
would be an updated version of Vernon Mark's initial treatment
of Leonard Kille, who suffered from attacks of rage. For three
months prior to performing a bilateral amygdalotomy on Kille,
Mark sent electric currents to the patient's brain via surgically
implanted depth electrodes, stimulating relaxed feelings and
apparently aborting his attacks.

A feedback system such as Ives envisions might also deliver

anticonvulsant drugs directly to the brain. "An internal monitor could note that the level of the anticonvulsant in the brain area where seizures usually start is dipping, and give a signal to release a small injection of the drug via an internal catheter," Ives says. While this technique has not yet been attempted on humans, researchers have stopped seizures in animals with anticonvulsant drugs. Since many TLE patients respond poorly to existing anticonvulsants, new epilepsy drugs are constantly being tested. In addition, doctors seek to understand why anticonvulsants sometimes help patients with manic-depressive illness or panic disorder, both of which may be seizure-based.

Future treatment of TLE may also depend more heavily on hormones, which may in turn benefit people with other hormone-related problems. According to Spiers, the eating disorders bulimia and anorexia may be caused by seizures. These seizures would most likely occur in the hypothalamus, a limbic structure connected to the pituitary gland that releases hormones involved in growth, temperature, cardiovascular function, sleep, thirst, and hunger. Also, since pregnancy reduces seizure frequency in some women, birth-control pills might be used to induce the hormonal equivalent of pregnancy in women with TLE. Furthermore, the high incidence of fertility problems in TLE patients may lead researchers to new treatments for infertility. And Spiers suspects that the common premenstrual syndrome, or PMS, consisting of strange tastes and moodiness that occurs only around the time of menstruation, is also a kind of epilepsy. "I bet that if you took one hundred women who have PMS and you did an EEG on them with special leads that could detect seizures anywhere in the brain," Spiers says, "fifty percent of them would have a seizure disorder around the time of menstruation." Doctors also hope to learn the reasons for improvement in the control of seizures in patients like Jill who make major life-style changes, such as giving up cigarettes, alcohol, or drugs, reducing stress, improving diet, and exercising regularly.

TLE holds forth promise in the quest to solve the mysteries of human behavior, but the answers it offers may ultimately be incomplete. There are limits to what we can know about the human brain, medicine's last frontier. In the twentieth century, we are beginning to make sense of it and to chart it. Molecular biology, physics, and neuropsychology give us ever better tools to examine the brain, while technology provides keener instruments with which to probe it, including lasers, electrodes, and computer-aided psychological tests. In the past half-century, evidence has accumulated about how neurons and neurotransmitters function. Yet the brain, like the atom, remains mostly a mystery. Like the atom, it seems to grow more complex as we home in on it. Because the brain is our tool for knowing the world, the distance between us and it can never be closed. We can never get outside ourselves to see the brain utterly, for it is itself our way of seeing.

Like the ancient concept of fate, TLE challenges the notion that one can willfully create the self. The disorder contributes to creativity, to violence, to Charlie's intellectual focus, and to Gloria's passionate anger, limiting the province of free will for good and for ill. It suggests that anatomy is destiny, as Freud once said, that personality is fixed, embedded in the structure and activity of the brain. The "Underground man" in Dostoevsky's *Notes from Underground* reaches a similar conclusion when in musing on his character he describes the "pleasure" that comes from the realization "that you no longer have any way out, that you will never become a different person; that even if there were still time and faith enough to change yourself, you probably would not even wish to change; and if you wished, you would do nothing about it anyway, because, in fact, there is perhaps nothing to change to." The same sense of personal stasis could result from an awareness of the self's dependence on the brain.

For Americans, whose culture is dependent on the notion that actions are largely volitional, this brain-mind link may be difficult to accept. After all, we are citizens of a nation nourished on the idea that each individual is the pioneer of a self with a boundless frontier. "Build your own world," Ralph Waldo Emerson exhorted. In the popular novels of Horatio Alger, newsboys and bootblacks attained wealth and success through simple virtues and hard work. The mottos of American society—Try Harder; Pull Yourself Up by Your Bootstraps; Every Man a King; Where There's a Will There's a Way—presume a tremendous amount of personal control. With our faith in the power of free will, we envision individuals creating, even remaking, themselves. We assume that we possess the fundamental power to determine the kind of person to be and how to behave. Although we accept that factors such as education, upbringing, and economic status play a role in determining character, we give free will the central role. The allure of this view is clear: it gives us a sense of control over our destinies and makes personal responsibility easy to assess. If we are good, according to this view, we deserve the credit. If we are bad, we deserve the blame.

But this view is too simple. It cannot explain people like van Gogh. Did he will his artwork or his suffering? His creativity or his suicide? If the answer is both, then who was in charge of the dual will that led him to such extremes? Were there two competing wills? If so, which will was truly free? TLE, a disorder of personal identity, of what Flaubert called his "me," challenges our assumption that we can control who we are and calls into question our conventional notions of credit and blame.

Because of TLE and other neuropsychiatric disorders, many neuroscientists and philosophers now see the mind-body distinction as illusory. The noted neuroscientist Roger Sperry, who has devoted his career to understanding the mind-body problem, concludes that mind and body are "inseparable parts of the same continuous hierarchy," two manifestations of a single reality. As the philosopher Gilbert Ryle put it, mind and matter are two aspects of one thing, related to each other in the way that team spirit is related to a team. Even Descartes, who wrote that "the mind by which I am what I am, is wholly distinct from the body," eventually rejected mind-body dualism and moved toward an understanding that psychological events have physical explanations. In his last work, *The Passions of the Soul*, published in 1649, a few weeks before he died, and still not widely read in English, Descartes acknowledged that mind and body are joined.

In Sperry's view, the notion that body and mind interact affects our concept of free will. "Human decision making," he writes, "is not indeterminant but self-determinant. Everyone normally wants to have control over what he does and to determine his own choices in accordance with his own wishes." Given the unity of body and mind, however, a person may be "relatively free" from "much that goes on around him, but he is not free from his own inner self." In a similar vein, the twentieth-century philosopher A. J. Ayer wrote, "The idea of the will as a piece of psychological mechanism which converts intentions into physical movements appears to be mythical. . . . The problems with which philosophers have vexed themselves . . . concerning the possibility of bridging the "gulf" between mind and matter . . . are all fictitious problems arising out of the senseless metaphysical conception of mind and matter . . . as 'substances.'" Ayer preferred to claim that human experiences "can be factually identified with states of the central nervous system. On this view, to have such and such an experience *is* for one's brain to be in such and such a state, in the way in which lightning *is* an electrical discharge. . . . This hypothesis may not be acceptable to those who wish to deny, in the interest of free-will, that human thoughts and actions are physically determined. . . . " But it is supported by "the very strong evidence of a general dependence of mental occurrences upon the functioning of the brain."

After observing that "we all limp, each to a greater or lesser degree," Dostoevsky's "Underground man" acknowledges our lust for personal control. "I know," he says, "that you may well get angry at me for these words, you may scold and stamp your feet: 'Talk about yourself and your underground miseries, but do not dare to say "*we all*."' But . . . I am by no means trying to justify myself by all this *we-allness*. As regards myself personally, I have in my own life merely carried to the extreme that which you have never ventured to carry even halfway. . . . So that, in fact, I may be even more 'alive' than you are." Like whatever mysterious force has caused this intensity in the "Underground man," TLE may compel people to carry "to the extreme" that which the rest of us never venture "to carry even halfway." Jill, for instance, now a sculptor, says that she feels more alive than ever before.

Like most of us, Jill is torn. She would like to believe that she has free will, but must acknowledge that TLE has changed who she is. The disorder has wrought both disadvantages and benefits. "TLE came at a bad time," she says. "It hit me in really important years. It played into and intensified the weaknesses and insecurities I already had, like the tendency to withdraw, to spend time by myself. Epilepsy kept me from getting close to people—men would say, 'I don't really know you,' because I always held myself back. When I felt sick, it was just easier to hold back. I'm not upset about the decisions I made. I'm not sure I wanted a committed relationship. I'm not sure I want to have a child. But the fact is that I didn't have the choice. The decision was not all in my hands." TLE limited her choices, but it also helped her to choose, by paving her way to art. In becoming a sculptor, Jill made a conscious decision to change occupations that is characteristic of her physical state. She is grateful to the disorder for having brought her to a new vocation. "TLE forced me to an extreme," she says, "to where I had to deal with myself and what I want to do."

Not long before she left her corporate job, she met a friend for dinner at a Chinese restaurant. The women talked about their lives, their health, and their plans. At the end of the meal, a waiter brought a plate of fortune cookies. Jill chose one, broke it, and silently read the message. "Here's a telling fortune," she said with a thoughtful smile: "We live not as we wish to, but as we can."

Selected Sources

Adams, Raymond D., and Maurice Victor. *Principles of Neurology*. 4th ed. New York: McGraw-Hill, 1989. Especially chap. 15, "Epilepsy and Other Seizure Disorders," and chap. 25, "The Limbic Lobes and the Neurology of Emotion."

Alajouanine, Théophile. "Dostoiewski's Epilepsy." *Brain* 86:209–218, 1963.

Allen, Hervey. *Israfel: The Life and Times of Edgar Allan Poe*. New York: George H. Doran, 1927.

Andreasen, Nancy C. *The Broken Brain: The Biological Revolution in Psychiatry*. New York: Harper & Row, 1984.

Anstett, Richard E., and Lorraine Wood. "The Patient Exhibiting Episodic Violent Behavior." *Journal of Family Practice* 16:605–609, 1983.

Armstrong, Karen. *Beginning the World*. New York: Macmillan, 1983.

Ayer, A. J. *The Central Questions of Philosophy*. London: Weidenfeld & Nicolson, 1973.

Bart, Benjamin F. *Flaubert*. Syracuse, N.Y.: Syracuse University Press, 1967.

Bass, Alison. "A Touch for Evil," profile of Dorothy Otnow Lewis. *Boston Globe Magazine*, 7 July 1991:12–26.

Bear, David M. "Hierarchical Neurology of Human Aggression." Paper presented at annual meeting of American Association for the Advancement of Science, Philadephia, May 1986.

―――. "The Neurology of Art: Artistic Creativity in Patients with Temporal Lobe Epilepsy." Paper presented at symposium "The Neurology of Art," Art Institute of Chicago and Michael Reese Hospital, Chicago, 1988.

―――. "The Significance of Behavioral Change in Temporal Lobe Epilepsy." *Journal of the McLean Hospital,* June 1977.

―――. "Temporal Lobe Epilepsy: A Syndrome of Sensory Limbic Hyperconnection." *Cortex* 15:357–384, 1979.

Bear, David, and Paul Fedio. "Quantitative Analysis of Interictal Behavior in Temporal Lobe Epilepsy." *Archives of Neurology* 34:454–467, 1977.

Bear, David M., Roy Freeman, David Schiff, and Mark Greenberg. "Interictal Behavior Changes in Patients with Temporal Lobe Epilepsy." *American Psychiatric Association Annual Review* 4, edited by R. E. Hales, and A. J. Frances, 1985.

Benson, D. F., and Dietrich Blumer, editors. *Psychiatric Aspects of Neurologic Disease.* New York: Grune & Stratton, 1975. Includes a chapter by Norman Geschwind on Dostoevsky's epilepsy.

Bercovitch, Sacvan. "The Myth of America." In *The Puritan Origins of the American Self.* New Haven: Yale University Press, 1975.

Bernstein, Richard. "The Electric Dreams of Philip K. Dick." *New York Times Book Review,* 3 November 1991:1, 30.

Bindra, Dalbir, with James A. Anderson, et al. *The Brain's Mind: A Neuroscience Perspective on the Mind-Body Problem.* New York: Gardner Press, 1980.

Blumer, Dietrich. "Hypersexual Episodes in Temporal Lobe Epilepsy." *American Journal of Psychiatry* 126:1099–1106, 1970.

―――. "A Profile of van Gogh from a Neuropsychiatric Point of View." Paper presented at symposium "The Neurology of Art," Art Institute of Chicago and Michael Reese Hospital, Chicago, 1988.

Blumer, Dietrich, editor. *Psychiatric Aspects of Epilepsy.* Washington, D.C.: American Psychiatric Association, 1984.

Blumer, Dietrich, and A. E. Walker. "Sexual Behavior in Temporal Lobe Epilepsy: A Study of the Effects of Temporal Lobectomy on Sexual Behavior." *Archives of Neurology* 16:37–43, 1967.

Bouchard, T. J., et al. "Sources of Human Psychological Differences: The Minnesota Study of Twins Reared Apart." *Science* 250:223–228, 1990.

Brandt, Frithiof. *Soren Kierkegaard*. Translated by Ann R. Born. Copenhagen: Det danske Selskab, 1963.

Browne, Thomas R., and Robert G. Feldman, editors. *Epilepsy: Diagnosis and Management*. Boston: Little, Brown, 1983.

Brownell, W. C. "Poe." In *American Prose Masters*, edited by H. M. Jones. Cambridge: Harvard University Press, 1963.

Bryant, John Ernest. *Genius and Epilepsy*. Concord, Mass.: Old Depot Press, 1953.

Camus, Albert. *L'Envers et l'Endroit*. Cambridge: Schoenhof, 1958. Preface.

Caplan, Lincoln. *The Insanity Defense and the Trial of John W. Hinckley, Jr.* New York: Dell, 1987.

Carpenter, Malcolm B. *Core Text of Neuroanatomy*, 2d ed. Baltimore: Williams & Wilkins, 1978.

Carroll, Lewis. *The Annotated Alice: Alice's Adventures in Wonderland & Through the Looking Glass*. Edited by Martin Gardner. New York: New American Library, 1960.

Catteau, Jacques. *Dostoyevsky and the Process of Literary Creation*. Translated by Audrey Littlewood. Cambridge, England: Cambridge University Press, 1989.

Chitty, Susan. *That Singular Person Called Lear: A Biography of Edward Lear, Artist, Traveler, and Prince of Nonsense*. New York: Atheneum, 1989.

Chorover, Stephan L. "Big Brother and Psychotechnology." *Psychology Today*, October 1973:43–54.

———. *From Genesis to Genocide: The Meaning of Human Nature and the Power of Behavior Control*. Cambridge, Mass.: MIT Press, 1979.

———. "Physician vs. Researcher: Values in Conflict?" *Wellesley*, Summer 1979:21–27.

———. "Psychosurgery: A Neuropsychological Perspective." *Boston University Law Review* 54:231–248, 1974.

Churchland, Patricia S. *Neurophilosophy: Toward a Unified Science of the Mind-Brain*. Cambridge, Mass.: MIT Press, 1986.

Chusid, Joseph G. *Correlative Neuroanatomy & Functional Neurology*, 15th ed. Los Altos, Calif.: Lange Medical Publications, 1973.

Cohen, Morton N., editor. *Lewis Carroll: Interviews and Recollections*. Iowa City: University of Iowa Press, 1989.

Cohen, Morton, and Roger Lancelyn Green. "Lewis Carroll's Loss of Consciousness." *Bulletin of the New York Public Library* 73:56–64, 1969.

Crichton, Michael. *The Terminal Man*. New York: Knopf, 1972.

Critchley, Macdonald. "Hughlings Jackson: The Sage of Manchester Square." In *The Citadel of the Senses*, New York: Raven Press, 1986.

———. "The Idea of a Presence." In *The Divine Banquet of the Brain and Other Essays*. New York: Raven Press, 1979.

Damasio, Antonio R., and Albert M. Galaburda. "Norman Geschwind." *Archives of Neurology* 42:500–504, 1985.

Davidson, Edward H. *Poe: A Critical Study*. Cambridge: Harvard University Press, 1957.

DeArmond, Stephen J., Madeline M. Fusco, and Maynard M. Dewey. *Structure of the Human Brain: A Photographic Atlas*, 2d ed. New York: Oxford University Press, 1976.

Descartes, René. *Discourse on Method*. Chicago: Paquin Printers, 1899.

———. *The Passions of the Soul*. Translated and annotated by Stephen Voss. Indianapolis: Hackett, 1989.

Devinsky, Orrin, and David Bear. "Varieties of Aggressive Behavior in Temporal Lobe Epilepsy." *American Journal of Psychiatry* 141:651–656, 1984.

Dewhurst, K., and A. W. Beard. "Sudden Religious Conversions in Temporal Lobe Epilepsy." *British Journal of Psychiatry* 117:497–507, 1970.

Dichter, Marc A. "The Epilepsies and Convulsive Disorders." Chap. 350 in *Harrison's Principles of Internal Medicine*, 12th ed., vol. 2. Edited by Jean D. Wilson et al. New York: McGraw-Hill, 1991.

Dick, Philip K. *Do Androids Dream of Electric Sheep?* New York: Ballantine, 1968.

———. *In Pursuit of Valis: Selections from the Exegesis*. Edited by Lawrence Sutin. Novato, Calif.: Underwood-Miller, 1991.

———. *The Three Stigmata of Palmer Eldritch*. London: Triad Grafton, 1978.

Disch, Thomas. "The Village Alien." *The Nation*, 14 March, 1987: 328–336.

Eccles, John, editor. *Mind and Brain: The Many-Faceted Problems*. Washington, D.C.: Paragon House, 1982.

Ellison, J. "Alterations of Sexual Behavior in Temporal Lobe Epilepsy." *Psychosomatics* 23:499–509, 1982.

Erickson, Kathleen Powers. "From Preaching to Painting: van Gogh's Religious Zeal." *The Christian Century* 107:300–302, 1990.

———. "Self-Portraits as Christ." *Bible Review* 6:24–31, 1990. Article based on "Van Gogh at Eternity's Gate: The Religious Aspects of

His Life and Work." Ph.D. diss. University of Chicago Divinity School.

Ewing, S. E. "'Absinthe Seizures': The Case of August Strindberg." Psychosomatic Conference, Department of Psychiatry, Mass. General Hospital, 25 September 1992.

Fields, William S., and William H. Sweet. *Neural Bases of Violence and Aggression.* St. Louis: W. H. Green, 1975.

Flaubert, Gustave. *The Letters of Gustave Flaubert 1830–1857.* Edited and translated by Francis Steegmuller. Cambridge, Mass.: Belknap/Harvard University Press, 1980–82.

Galaburda, Albert M. "Norman Geschwind 1926–1984." *Neuropsychologia* 23:297–304, 1985.

Galvin, Ruth Mehrtens. "The Nature of Shyness." *Harvard Magazine,* March/April 1992:40–45.

Gardner, Howard. *The Shattered Mind.* New York: Random House, 1974.

Gastaut, Henri. "Fyodor Mikhailovitch Dostoyevsky's Involuntary Contribution to the Symptomatology and Prognosis of Epilepsy." *Epilepsia* 19:186–201, 1978.

———. "Mémoires Originaux: La Maladie de Vincent van Gogh envisagée à la lumière des conceptions nouvelles sur l'epilepsie psychomotrice." *Annales medico-psychologiques* 114:196–238, 1956.

Gastaut, Henri, and Y. Gastaut. "La Maladie de Gustave Flaubert." *Révue neurologique* 138:467–492, 1982.

Gazzaniga, Michael. *Mind Matters: How Mind and Brain Interact to Create Our Conscious Lives.* Boston: Houghton-Mifflin, 1988.

Gazzaniga, Michael, editor. *Handbook of Cognitive Neuroscience.* New York: Plenum Press, 1984.

Geschwind, Norman. "Behavioral Change in Temporal Lobe Epilepsy." *Archives of Neurology* 34:453, 1977.

———. "Behavioural Changes in Temporal Lobe Epilepsy." *Psychological Medicine* 9:217, 1979.

———. "Epilepsy in the Life and Writings of Dostoievsky." Lecture given at Boston Society of Psychiatry and Neurology, March 16, 1961.

———. "Interictal Behavioral Changes in Epilepsy." *Epilepsia* 24:523–530, 1983.

———. "Left-handedness: Association with Immune Disease, Migraine, and Developmental Learning Disorder." *Proceedings of the National Academy of Sciences, U.S.A.* 79:5097–5100, 1982.

Geschwind, Norman, and Albert M. Galaburda, editors. *Cerebral Dominance: The Biological Foundations.* Cambridge: Harvard University Press, 1984.

Gibb, H. A., and J. H. Kramers. *Shorter Encyclopaedia of Islam.* Ithaca, N.Y.: Cornell University Press, 1957.

Gibbs, Frederic A. "Ictal and Non-ictal Psychiatric Disorders in Temporal Lobe Epilepsy." *Journal of Nervous and Mental Disease* 113:522–528, 1951.

Gilbert, Judson B., and Gordon E. Mestler. *Disease and Destiny: A Bibliography of Medical References to the Famous.* London: Dawsons of Pall Mall, 1962.

Gloor, Pierre, et al. "The Role of the Limbic System in Experiential Phenomena of Temporal Lobe Epilepsy." *Annals of Neurology* 12: 129–144, 1982.

Gogh, Vincent van. *Dear Theo: The Autobiography of Vincent van Gogh.* Edited by Irving Stone. New York: Doubleday, 1937.

————. *The Letters of Vincent van Gogh.* Edited by Mark Roskill. London: Fontana, 1983.

Goleman, Daniel. "When Rage Explodes, Brain Damage May Be the Cause." *New York Times,* 7 August 1990. C1.

Goodglass, Harold. "Norman Geschwind (1926–1984)." *Cortex* 22:7–10, 1986.

Gotman, Jean, John R. Ives, and Pierre Gloor. *Long-Term Monitoring in Epilepsy.* Amsterdam, the Netherlands: Elsevier Science Publishers, 1985.

Graetz, H. R. *The Symbolic Language of Vincent van Gogh.* New York: McGraw-Hill, 1963.

Green, Joseph B., editor. *Neurologic Clinics* 2 (1):1–175, 1984. Symposium on Borderland Between Neurology and Psychiatry.

Hansen, Heidi, and L. Bork Hansen, "The Temporal Lobe Epilepsy Syndrome Elucidated Through Soren Kierkegaard's Authorship and Life." *Acta Psychiatr. Scand.* 77:352–358, 1988.

Hecaen, Henri, and Martin L. Albert. *Human Neuropsychology.* New York: Wiley, 1978.

Herzog, Andrew, et al. "Neuroendocrine Dysfunction in Temporal Lobe Epilepsy." *Archives of Neurology* 39:133–135, 1982.

————. "Reproductive Endocrine Disorders in Men with Partial Seizures of Temporal Lobe Origin." *Archives of Neurology* 43:347–350, 1986.

————. "Reproductive Endocrine Disorders in Women with Partial

Seizures of Temporal Lobe Origin." *Archives of Neurology* 43:341–346, 1986.

———. "Temporal Lobe Epilepsy: An Extrahypothalamic Pathogenesis for Polycystic Ovarian Syndrome?" *Neurology* 34:1389–1393, 1984.

Hingley, Ronald. *Dostoyevsky, His Life and Work.* New York: Charles Scribner's Sons, 1978.

Hoffman, Daniel. *Poe Poe Poe Poe Poe Poe Poe Poe.* New York: Doubleday, 1972.

Hubel, David H. "The Brain." *Scientific American* 241(3):44–53, 1979.

Hunt, Joe. "Politics of Psychosurgery." *The Real Paper* 2 (22), 30 May 1973:6–10.

Inman, Arthur C. *The Inman Diary: A Public and Private Confession.* Two volumes. Edited by Daniel Aaron. Cambridge: Harvard University Press, 1985.

Jackson, J. Hughlings. *Neurological Fragments,* with biographical memoir by James Taylor. London: Oxford University Press, 1925.

James, William. *The Varieties of Religious Experience.* New York: Macmillan, 1961.

Kaplan, Edith, and Dean C. Delis. "The Neuropsychology of '10 After 11': A Qualitative Analysis of Clock Drawings by Brain-Damaged Patients." In *Clock Drawings: A Neuropsychology Analysis,* edited by M. Freedman et al. New York: Oxford University Press, in press.

Khoshbin, Shahram. "Clinical Neurophysiology of Aggressive Behavior." Paper presented at annual meeting of the American Association for the Advancement of Science, Philadelphia, May 1986.

———. "What Really Was van Gogh's Malady?" *Perspectives,* Winter 1986:6–7. Publication of Harvard Medical School, Boston.

Klüver, Heinrich, and Paul C. Bucy. "Preliminary Analysis of Functions of the Temporal Lobes in Monkeys." *Archives of Neurology and Psychiatry* 42:979–1000, 1939.

———. "'Psychic Blindness' and Other Symptoms Following Bilateral Temporal Lobectomy in Rhesus Monkeys." *American Journal of Physiology* 119:352–353, 1937.

Landsborough, David. "St. Paul and Temporal Lobe Epilepsy." *Journal of Neurology, Neurosurgery, & Psychiatry* 50:659–664, 1987.

LaPlante, Eve. "The Riddle of TLE." *The Atlantic,* November 1988:30–35.

Lassek, Arthur M. *The Unique Legacy of Doctor Hughlings Jackson.* Springfield, Ill.: Charles C. Thomas, 1970.

Lawall, John. "Psychiatric Presentations of Seizure Disorders." *American Journal of Psychiatry* 133:321–323, 1976.

Lechtenberg, Richard. *Epilepsy and the Family.* Cambridge: Harvard University Press, 1984.

Lennox, William Gordon, with Margaret A. Lennox. *Epilepsy and Related Disorders.* Two volumes. Boston: Little, Brown, 1960.

Lewis, Dorothy Otnow, et al. "Psychomotor Epilepsy and Violence in a Group of Incarcerated Adolescent Boys." *American Journal of Psychiatry* 139:882–887, 1982.

Lewis, Dorothy Otnow, Jonathan H. Pincus, and Melvin Lewis. "Psychomotor Symptoms, Psychotic Episodes, Physical Abuse, and Family Violence: A Limbic Psychotic Aggressive Syndrome." Paper presented at annual meeting of American Association for the Advancement of Science, Philadelphia, May 1986.

Lewis, Jefferson. *Something Hidden: A Biography of Wilder Penfield.* Toronto: Doubleday, 1981.

Lockard, Joan S., and Arthur A. Ward, Jr. *Epilepsy: A Window to Brain Mechanisms.* New York: Raven Press, 1980.

Lottman, Herbert. *Flaubert: A Biography.* Boston: Little, Brown, 1989.

Lubin, Albert J. *Stranger on the Earth: A Psychological Biography of Vincent van Gogh.* New York: Holt, Rinehart & Winston, 1972.

Luria, A. R. *The Working Brain: An Introduction to Neuropsychology.* New York: Basic Books, 1973.

Mark, Vernon, and Frank R. Ervin. *Violence and the Brain.* New York: Harper & Row, 1970.

Martin, Robert Bernard. *Tennyson: The Unquiet Heart.* New York: Oxford University Press, 1980.

Mayer, André, and Michael Wheeler. *The Crocodile Man: A Case of Brain Chemistry and Criminal Violence.* Boston: Houghton Mifflin, 1982.

Mesulam, M-Marsel, editor. *Principles of Behavioral Neurology.* Philadelphia: F. A. Davis, 1985. See especially chap. 8, "Temporolimbic Epilepsy and Behavior."

Monroe, Russell R. *Episodic Behavioral Disorders: A Psychodynamic and Neurophysiologic Analysis.* Cambridge: Harvard University Press, 1970.

———. "Limbic Ictus and Atypical Psychoses." *Journal of Nervous and Mental Disease* 170:711–716, 1982.

Morley, T. P., editor. *Current Controversies in Neurosurgery.* Philadelphia: W. B. Saunders, 1976.

Muir, Sir William. *Life of Mohammad.* Edinburgh: Grant, 1923.

Mumenthaler, Mark. *Neurology,* 2d ed. New York: Thieme-Stratton, 1983.

Mungas, Dan. "An Empirical Analysis of Specific Syndromes of Violent Behavior." *Journal of Nervous and Mental Disease* 171:354–361, 1983.

Nadis, Steve. "Angels from the Temporal Lobe." Unpublished manuscript, Cambridge, 1990.

Nicholi, Armand M., Jr., editor. *New Harvard Guide to Psychiatry.* Cambridge: Belknap/Harvard University Press, 1988.

Nolte, John. *The Human Brain: An Introduction to Its Functional Anatomy.* St. Louis: C. V. Mosby, 1981.

Overman, Brenda F. *Wellbeing.* November 1984. Publication of Beth Israel Hospital, Boston.

Penfield, Wilder. *The Mystery of the Mind: A Critical Study of Consciousness and the Human Brain.* Princeton: Princeton University Press, 1975.

Penfield, Wilder, and T. Rasmussen. *The Cerebral Cortex of Man.* New York: Macmillan, 1950.

Penfield, Wilder, and Theodore C. Erickson. *Epilepsy and Cerebral Localization.* Springfield, Ill: Charles C. Thomas, 1941.

Penfield, Wilder, and H. H. Jasper. *Epilepsy and the Functional Anatomy of the Human Brain.* Boston: Little, Brown, 1954.

Percy, Walker. *The Second Coming.* New York: Farrar, Straus, Giroux, 1980.

———. *The Thanatos Syndrome.* New York: Farrar, Straus, Giroux, 1987.

Persinger, Michael A. "People Who Report Religious Experiences May Also Display Enhanced Temporal-Lobe Signs." *Perceptual & Motor Skills* 58:963–975, 1984.

———. "Religious and Mystical Experiences as Artifacts of Temporal Lobe Function: A General Hypothesis." *Perceptual & Motor Skills* 57:1255–1262, 1983.

———. "Striking EEG Profiles from Single Episodes of Glossolalia and Transcendental Meditation." *Perceptual & Motor Skills* 58:127–133, 1984.

Persinger, Michael A., and K. Makarec. "Temporal Lobe Epileptic Signs and Correlative Behaviors Displayed by Normal Populations." *Journal of General Psychology* 114:179–195, 1987.

Pickvance, Ronald. *Van Gogh in Arles.* New York: Metropolitan Museum of Art, 1984.

———. *Van Gogh in Saint-Rémy and Auvers.* New York: Metropolitan Museum of Art, 1986.

Pines, Maya. *The Brain Changers: Scientists and the New Mind Control.* New York: Harcourt Brace Jovanovich, 1973.

Poe, Edgar Allan. *The Complete Tales and Poems of Edgar Allan Poe.* Introduced by Hervey Allen. New York: Modern Library, 1965.

Pollack, Richard. *The Episode.* New York: New American Library, 1986.

Pollock, Daniel C. "The Kindling Model as a Means of Understanding Aggressive Behavior." Paper presented at annual meeting of American Association for the Advancement of Science, Philadelphia, May 1986.

Popper, Karl R., and John C. Eccles. *The Self and Its Brain.* New York: Springer International, 1977.

Priestland, Gerald. *The Case Against God.* London: Collins, 1984.

Pritchett, V. S., editor. "Lewis Carroll: Letters." In *A Man of Letters: Selected Essays.* New York: Random House, 1985.

Reiser, Morton F., editor. *Organic Disorders and Psychosomatic Medicine.* Vol. 4 of *American Handbook of Psychiatry,* 2d ed. New York: Basic Books, 1975.

Remillard, G. M., et al. "Sexual Ictal Manifestations Predominate in Women with Temporal Lobe Epilepsy: A Finding Suggesting Sexual Dimorphism in the Human Brain." *Neurology* 33:323–330, 1983.

Reynolds, Edward H. "Hughlings Jackson: A Yorkshireman's Contribution to Epilepsy." *Archives of Neurology* 45:675–678, 1988.

Rice, James L. *Dostoevsky and the Healing Art: An Essay in Literary and Medical History.* Ann Arbor, Mich.: Ardis, 1985.

Rickman, Gregg. "Introduction to 'The Riddle of TLE.'" *Philip K. Dick Society Newsletter* 20:3–4, 1989.

Rise, Matthew L., et al. "Genes for Epilepsy Mapped in the Mouse." *Science* 253:669–673, 1991.

Rosenfield, Israel. "A Hero of the Brain." Review of Norman Geschwind's work. *New York Review of Books,* 21 November 1985:49–55.

Ryle, Gilbert. *The Concept of Mind.* Chicago: University of Chicago Press, 1949.

Sachdev, H. S., and Stephen G. Waxman. "Frequency of Hypergraphia in Temporal Lobe Epilepsy: An Index of Interictal Behaviour Syndrome." *Journal of Neurology, Neurosurgery, and Psychiatry* 44:358–360, 1981.

Sacks, Oliver. *The Man Who Mistook His Wife for a Hat and Other Clinical Tales.* New York: Harper & Row, 1987.

Schweitzer, Albert. *The Mysticism of Saint Paul.* London: Adam & Charles Black, 1967.

Sheer, Daniel E., editor. *Electrical Stimulation of the Brain.* Austin, Tex.: University of Texas Press, 1961.

Slater, Eliot, et al. "The Schizophrenia-like Psychoses of Epilepsy." *British Journal of Psychiatry* 109:95–150, 1963.

Sperry, Roger W. "Mind-Brain Interaction: Mentalism, Yes; Dualism, No." *Neuroscience* 5:195–206, 1980.

———. *Science and Moral Priority: Merging Mind, Brain, and Human Values.* New York: Columbia University Press, 1983.

Spinoza, Baruch. *The Ethics and Selected Letters.* Translated by Samuel Shirley; edited by Seymour Feldman. Indianapolis, Ind.: Hackett, 1982.

Spong, John Shelby. *Rescuing the Bible from Fundamentalism.* New York: HarperCollins, 1991.

Stern, Theodore A., and George B. Murray. "Complex Partial Seizures Presenting as a Psychiatric Illness." *Journal of Nervous & Mental Disease* 172:625–627, 1984.

Stevens, Janice R., and Bruce P. Hermann. "Temporal Lobe Epilepsy, Psychopathology, and Violence: The State of the Evidence." *Neurology* 31:1127–1132, 1981.

Strieber, Whitley. *Communion: A True Story.* New York: William Morrow, 1987.

Sutin, Lawrence. *Divine Invasions: A Life of Philip K. Dick.* New York: Crown, 1989.

Sweetman, David. *Van Gogh: His Life and His Art.* New York: Crown, 1990.

Taylor, D. C. "Sexual Behavior and Temporal Lobe Epilepsy." *Archives of Neurology* 21:510–516, 1969.

Temkin, Owsei. *The Falling Sickness.* Baltimore: Johns Hopkins Press, 1971.

Terzian, Hrayr, and G. Dalle Ore. "Syndrome of Klüver and Bucy Reproduced in Man by Bilateral Removal of the Temporal Lobes." *Neurology* 5:373–380, 1955.

Tomkins, Calvin. "A Reporter at Large: Irises." *The New Yorker,* 4 April 1988:37–67.

Treiman, D. M. "Epilepsy and Violence: Medical and Legal Issues." *Epilepsia* 27 suppl. 2:S77–S104, 1986.

Trimble, Michael R. *Epilepsy, Behaviour, and Cognitive Function.* London: Wiley, 1988.

Trimble, Michael R., and T. G. Bolwig, editors. *Aspects of Epilepsy and Psychiatry.* London: Wiley, 1986.

Valenstein, Elliot S. *Great and Desperate Cures: The Rise and Decline of Psychosurgery and Other Radical Treatments for Mental Illness*. New York: Basic Books, 1986.

———. *The Psychosurgery Debate: Scientific, Legal, and Ethical Perspectives*. San Francisco: Freeman, 1980.

Valeo, Tom. "A Glimpse of How Mind Produces Art." *Boston Globe* 16 January 1989:45.

Wallace, Richard. *The Agony of Lewis Carroll*. Melrose, Mass.: Gemini Press, 1990.

Ward, A. A., Jr., et al., editors. *Epilepsy*. New York: Raven Press, 1983.

Waxman, Stephen G., and Norman Geschwind. "Hypergraphia in Temporal Lobe Epilepsy." *Neurology* 24:629–636, 1974.

———. "The Interictal Behavior Syndrome Associated with Temporal Lobe Epilepsy." *Archives of General Psychiatry* 32:1580–1586, 1975.

Whitman, Steven G., and Bruce P. Hermann. *Psychopathology in Epilepsy: Social Dimensions*. New York: Oxford University Press, 1986.

Williams, Denis. "The Structure of Emotions Reflected in Epileptic Experience." *Brain* 79:29–67, 1956.

———. "Temporal Lobe Epilepsy." *British Medical Journal* 1:1439–1442, 1966.

Winnicott, D. W. *The Spontaneous Gesture*. Cambridge: Harvard University Press, 1987.

Acknowledgments

This book is the result of numberless false starts, chance meetings, and casual conversations over more than seven years, so I have many people to thank. I am grateful to the three extraordinary "ordinary people" with TLE who opened their personal and medical histories to me, and to the numerous physicians and psychologists who appear in the book.

Other people who directly or indirectly contributed to the book include Dr. Martin Albert, Michael Aronson, Dr. Sheldon Benjamin, Sacvan Bercovitch, Dr. Howard Blume, Tom and Caroline Bridgman Rees, Rodney Brisco, Dr. Rachel Buchsbaum, Debra Cash, Emer bean i Chuiv, Hunter Corbett, Dr. David Coulter, Peter Crino, Andrew Dreyfus, Carl Dreyfus, Mary Elliot, Dr. Albert England, Donald Fanger, Dr. Robert Feldman, Dr. Annie Fine, Frances Conover Fitch, the late Dr. Stuart Flerlage, Kent French, Kimberly French, Angel Garcia, Howard Gardner, Sheila Gillooly, Laura Goldin, David Goodman, Tom Kiely, Mark Kramer, Deanie LaPlante, Jane Larsen, Steve Linsky, Eleanor Lowry, Alison McGandy, Dr. Jamin McMahon, Patrick McNamara, Eugene and Joanne Mallove, Bill Mellins, Dr. James Morris, Steve Nadis, Margaret O'Donnell, Diana Raffman, Nancy Raffman, Rita Raffman, John Rasmussen, Alice Rosengard, Norma Santamaria, Israel Scheffler, Patricia Osborne Shafer, Barbara and Paul Simkowski, Anne

Squire, Rick Summers, and George Viglirolo. I am also grateful to reporter Jean Dietz and editor Harry King, formerly of the *Boston Globe;* Dr. Marlene Oscar Berman and Dr. Edith Kaplan of the Boston University School of Medicine; and Daniel Aaron and Libby Smith, editors of the Inman diary. The staffs of the Houghton Library at Harvard University, the Epilepsy Foundation of Boston, and the Epilepsy Foundation of America provided helpful information.

For special assistance I wish to thank Gerry Deeney, Sandy Fowler, Glenn Gibbs, Betty Green, and Elaine Soffer. I am grateful to C. Michael Curtis for his early faith, and to John McPhee, Susan Sheehan, and E. B. White for the examples they set. Donald W. Thomas of Brookline High School gave me a teaching job and much more. In suffering from neurological disease, my father, Joseph A. LaPlante, was an early muse; to my regret he did not live to read the finished book. Virginia W. LaPlante, my mother, edited countless drafts and shared every glitch and triumph along the way. My husband, David M. Dorfman, provided support and advice, and as I honed the book he listened to every word. I am grateful to Rick Kot, my editor, for his unerring judgment, and, finally, to my agent, Sallie Gouverneur, for her gentle encouragement and editorial insight.

Index